BRAIN FITNESS for WOMEN

BRAIN

FITNESS

for *WOMEN*

Keeping Your Head Clear & Your Mind Sharp at Any Age

SONDRA KORNBLATT

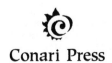

Conari Press

First published in 2012 by Conari Press, an imprint of
Red Wheel/Weiser, LLC
With offices at:
665 Third Street, Suite 400
San Francisco, CA 94107
www.redwheelweiser.com

ISBN: 978-1-57324-490-9

Library of Congress Cataloging-in-Publication Data

Kornblatt, Sondra.
    Brain fitness for women : keeping your head clear and your mind sharp at any age /
Sondra Kornblatt.
        p. cm.
    Summary: "Did you know that women have 70,000 thoughts per day and one per-
son's brain generates more electrical impulses each day than all the telephones in the
world combined?In Brain Fitness for Women, health writer Sondra Kornblatt offers an
entertaining look at how women's brains work: the physiology of women's brains, new
research in neuroscience, the differences between women's and men's brains, and how
women's brains age. Kornblatt offers fun facts (yep, that chocolate you're craving does
boost cognitive function), tips (your brain wants a glass of water in the morning), and
advice (forget multitasking, the brain can only process one thing at a time) for women
who want to keep their minds in tiptop shape. She examines how hormones, the environment, exercise, stress, food, aging, and even friendship affect the brain, and offers
strategies for keeping your brain on its metaphorical tiptoes at any age"-- Provided by
publisher.
    Includes bibliographical references and index.
    ISBN 978-1-57324-490-9 (pbk.)
    1. Brain--Sex differences. 2. Women--Health and hygiene. I. Title.
    QP376.K655 2011
    612.8'2082--dc23
                                                    2011036141

Cover design by Nita Ybarra
Interior by Jane Hagaman
Typeset in Bembo and Bulmer MT Std

Printed in the United States of America
QG
10 9 8 7 6 5 4 3 2 1

To Milo and Ella for patience, flexibility, and independence

*To my parents David and Barbara for love, support,
and their perpetual willingness to learn*

Contents

Foreword

Medical school professors who have a sense of history will sometimes tell their students that half of what they are learning is wrong—but that we don't yet know which half that will turn out to be. Medical knowledge has been evolving and changing for a long time, whether or not its teachers knew it (or would admit it). In the fourth century BCE, Aristotle thought that the seat of intelligence was in the heart. The blood carried the hot emotions, and the role of the brain was to cool it. Human brains cooled more than smaller animal brains did, making humans more rational. That's not the way we think the brain works today.

Now, fast-forward almost up to the present. As a medical student, I recall reading an old article on the neuroanatomical basis of emotion and memory. This article has stood the test of time: it laid the foundation upon which our current understanding of this area is based. I was shocked, however, to find a sentence in it which would not have made it past the scientific reviewers even in my school days- saying, in effect, that "We don't know what this part of the brain does, but since it's bigger in men than in women we assume it must have something to do with sex."

If all this isn't enough of a challenge, there's also the problem of how fast new information accumulates. When I was in college many years ago, one of my chemistry professors described a study which had been done to look at the production of new information in the field. It concluded that if someone spent forty hours a week doing nothing but reading the new scientific literature as it was published, by the end of the year she would be months behind! Today's diligent scientist would undoubtedly fare even worse.

We're bombarded all the time with news of breakthroughs and new theories about how to improve our health. Unfortunately, many of these result in conflicting advice. Is hormone replacement therapy good or bad? What about caffeine? Should I take supplements, or not? Eat butter or margarine? How much red wine should I drink with my fish? Is it safe to eat the apples yet? Will my cell phone give me brain cancer?

You don't have to go to medical school and read ponderous scientific journals all day to find a path through this heap of information. In this book, Sondra Kornblatt will guide you through it. She explains how the brain is put together, how it works, and how it influences many aspects of your life. You'll learn how it produces moods and emotions and how hormones affect it. You'll gain practical tips about supporting your brain: how to feed it, rest it, amuse it, help it repair itself, and keep it healthy. You'll learn about sleep, exercise, and diet; vitamins, supplements, and toxins; meditation and clever tricks for remembering things; and even the benefits of "yawn attacks." You'll have some laughs—and that is also good for your brain.

This book is well-researched and presents current brain science in a comprehensible way. The information here is practical and comes from both Western medical and alternative viewpoints. You don't have to be a doctor or neuroscientist to benefit from it. In thirty years as a neurologist, I've seen women of all ages who are concerned about their brain health. This book is a wonderful tool for anyone who wants to understand how to keep her brain happy and functioning at its peak for a very long time.

Jean Millican, MD
Seattle, Washington

Acknowledgments

Writing this book was like making a clay sculpture. I had to search the earth for clay, dig it, mix it, wedge it, envision it, shape it, smash it down, reshape it, simplify it, and finally glaze and fire it.

It wasn't a lonely journey. My caring community of family and friends helped me from the search for clay to the kiln. They kept me from trashing the book, my sanity, and my brain.

A bounty of appreciation to my editor, Caroline Pincus, associate publisher at Conari Press, for wise edits delivered with kindness; Susie Pitzen; Robin Doyle, who also reviewed the manuscript and made excellent suggestions; and marketing at Red Wheel/Weiser and Conari Press for being the best book people; my parents group, PEPS (Program for Early Parent Support), which has supported, fed, and loved my family for nineteen years; my Communications Department cadre who meet the challenges of Group Health with as much sanity and as little jargon as possible; Sasha London, for research and assistance; Rebecca Parsons, for humor, editing, and good hair advice; Ella Hansen, for nonpareil citations; Ragini Michaels, for reminding me of the book's vision and teaching me to be more present in this paradoxical life; and Howard, Diane, and Michael, for the support that lasts.

And mostly to my children: Milo and Ella, thank you for your writing opinions, grocery shopping, *Glee* watching, music sharing, Sadie loving, dish wrangling, and dinner celebrations. Let me know what you think if you ever read this book. I love you.

Chapter 1

The Weary Brain

A brain is a lot like a computer. It will only take so many facts,
and then it will go on overload and blow up.

Erma Bombeck, humorist

Women are overloaded.

Need proof? Look at the covers of magazines in the grocery line for the long list of things we "should" attend to.

Lose 11 pounds in 7 days. Exfoliate your skin. Buy the latest fashions. Get a flat stomach. Organize your garage. Six tips to get ahead at work. Save for retirement. Latest smart investments. Five sexy ways to make your man love you. Eat right for your unborn baby. Parenting the terrible twos. Help your children read in just ten minutes a day. Get your teens to church. Find your best new smart phone. Beware of toxins in your furniture. Choose the right Botox doctor. When to bikini wax in the winter. Cook healthy quick meals. Build a compost bin. Care for your mother across the country. Stay fit through all ages.

We're living in a world so fast paced, with so many expectations, it's really crazy. There's a limit to what the nervous system can handle, and most of us are way over the limit.[1] With demands coming from all sides, we feel like we're going to lose our minds—and perhaps our brains too.

Your brain is the center of your stormy life, but it is not like the quiet, calm eye of a hurricane. Your brain is more like a boat in a harbor, whipped around in winds and cross currents, banging against the pier, held by ropes that are straining against the stress.

You can hear it in your language: you say you forgot a parent-teacher conference because of *brain fog*, missed a party because you were *brain fried,* can't retrieve the name of a book author because of a *brain fart,* or procrastinate learning a new telephone system at work because your *brain is toast.*

Poor brain. It has to orchestrate everything: muscles, hormones, digestion, mood, speech, sleep, memory, dreams, compassion, emotions, actions, and stress.

Even though it's doing all that, it's easy to take the brain for granted. You frequently don't give yourself the things your brain needs to function well: good foods, exercise, stimulating challenges, a nontoxic environment, quiet time, nature, bigger perspectives, emotional care, friends to talk with, and respect for what it's doing.

There's only so much you can change outside, but you can change what you do, including how you support the brain.

Taking care of your brain can change your life.

You and your brain need care to stay sane in this crazy world. When you support your brain, it has more resources to handle what's expected of it. You'll be more relaxed about your overwhelming to-do lists. You'll also know how to stop blaming yourself and your brain for not handling the impossible. Instead, you'll support your brain in order to get the best from it—and from your life.

Brain Fitness for Women shows you holistic ways to sustain your brain—more than just clever games that stretch your cognitive ability, like most brain-fitness books focus on. Your cognitive ability is just one part of your brain, and there are many factors that influence our brains every day: toxins, information overload, overwhelming emotions, and hormone changes.

You'll learn what revives the brain, including exercising, volunteering, socializing, and spending time in nature. *Brain Fitness for Women* shares the latest on the brain and food choices, learning, memory help, and meditation. You'll also read about:

- Triggering biophelia (attraction to nature) in your house;
- Myths about male and female brains, and what really makes them different;
- Myths about preventing Alzheimer's and what really helps;

- Toxins in your cosmetics and how to avoid them;
- How both movement and stillness improve your brain.

Some techniques may be new to you; some you may have forgotten. Some may be small steps; some may be big leaps. In all cases, the aim is to help you form a new relationship with your brain—and your life.

This book will help you appreciate and love the miracle under your skull, one that extends via communication systems throughout your body to the tips of your fingers and toes. Treat yourself and your brain in the same way you would a new love on your first dates—good dinner, stimulating activities, long walks, and quiet moments just being together.

When you care for your brain using the tips in this book, you will support how it functions, understand its human limitations, and foster a long and healthy partnership with your unique genius. (And happily, all the ways that support the brain also support the body.) The best part of your brilliant neural phenomenon: despite all the ups and downs, it can be grateful for the blessing of being alive.

So let's turn away from the headlines in those women's magazines and learn how to revive our brains and make them fit for us, in all dimensions.

Chapter 2

Brain Basics
Does Your Brain Know It's a Girl?

*With modern parts atop old ones, the brain is like
an iPod built around an eight-track cassette player.*

Sharon Begley, journalist

*If a woman has to choose between catching a fly ball
and saving an infant's life, she will chose to save the infant's life
without even considering if there are men on base.*

Dave Barry, humorist

By the time my daughter was eight, she was pretty blasé when people mistook her for a boy, which was a fairly common occurrence. After all, my daughter usually wore a baseball (not softball) uniform or comfortable clothes from the boys' department—not pink or purple clothes with short, useless sleeves and lace. Her hair was short, her style was brisk, and it was perfectly logical that sales clerks, strangers in the park, and even new parents at school would assume she was a boy.

Even though it wasn't easy for strangers to tell that my daughter was a girl, she knew she was one. And even though it's not easy to tell if a young brain (in a lab, without the body) belongs to a boy or girl, the brain knows what it is—at least as far as basic reproduction. Beyond that, there are plenty of questions and plenty of opinions about whether our actions are hardwired into the gender of the brain.

We'll look at the brain and sex in this chapter and the next, after we understand a little bit about the miracle everyone has inside their skull.

The Basic Brain

The brain is the most complex structure on earth.[2] The physical brain—consisting of mostly water (about 78%), plus fats, proteins, and carbohydrates—can sense the outside and inner world, create thoughts and feelings, keep you breathing and pumping blood, and discover new ways to relate to the world. The brain is mind-boggling.

To understand the components of the awesome brain, let's create a model using your hands. Make two fists, touching the first knuckles together and keeping your thumbs parallel. Your combined fists are about the size of a brain.

Now, imagine that between your fists is a ball of bread dough about the size of a tennis ball; inside the dough are two shelled almonds and two shelled walnuts, one of each within the dough in either fist. This dough is your *limbic* system, the oldest part of your brain; it supports basic brain functions, including emotion, behavior, and long-term memory. The two almonds together are your *amygdalae,* which govern your emotions and fight-or-flight fear response. The two walnuts represent your *thalamus,* the center for sensory and motor functions.

Now bend your arms so your elbows point to the floor and your knuckles point to the sky. If someone put a pencil between your arms, that pencil would be your spinal cord, and your wrists would be your *brain stem.* The brain stem manages basic body functions, such as heart rate and consciousness (being awake or sleepy). Combine the limbic system and brain stem (the dough ball and your wrists), and you have a pretty functional brain system for animals.

But we're missing the *cerebellum,* which you can imagine as a big blob of dough squeezed out of the back, or pinky side, of your hand, by your wrist. The cerebellum is called a "little brain." It's like a little computer that connects and coordinates motor control, cognitive functions such as attention and language, and probably some emotional responses such as fear and pleasure. The cerebellum connects to the more complex *cerebral cortex* on top of the brain.[3]

Your combined fists represent the two hemispheres of the *cerebrum* and their fissures (folds that increase the surface area of the brain).

The thumb side is the front of the brain: the *frontal lobes* responsible for reasoning, motivation, and other higher brain functions that allow you to read, drive, and play Wii Fit. The middle fingers are the *parietal lobes,* which are responsible for touch, movement, and orientation. The backs of the hands (nearest the ears in a person, if the brain were in a head) are the *temporal lobes,* responsible for auditory stimuli, memory, and speech. Finally, the pinky fingers are the *occipital lobes,* responsible for visual processing.[4]

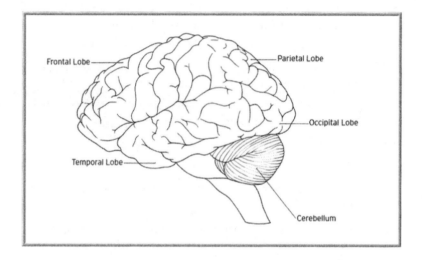

You've got the whole world in your hands. But beyond this basic view are many more ways to slice and analyze the brain.

A Universe of Neurons

The field of neuroscience is now being compared with astronomy, because they both deal with unknowns of similar magnitude. You know how you feel the infinite expanse of the universe when you see a thick carpet of stars in a dark sky? That magnitude is echoed in our brains, which hold hundreds of trillions of synapses—1,500 times the number of stars that fill the Milky Way galaxy.

> *Our brains have hundreds of trillions of synapses—*
> *1,500 times the number of stars in the Milky Way galaxy.*

Information travels quickly in our brains—very quickly. The *slowest* speed that information is transferred between neurons is 260 mph. That's slightly faster than the speed of the original Bugatti EB, one of the fastest road-legal cars in the world, clocked at 253 mph.

Our brains are not only fast, but also busy. One human brain has an average of 70,000 thoughts per day and generates more electrical impulses than all the telephones in the world combined.

The most obvious magical marvels that do all this work are called **neurons,** the primary cells of our brain and nervous system. About 100 billion neurons live under your skull in your three-pound spongy ball of brilliance. Each neuron looks like a spindly tree drawn by Dr. Seuss and consists of three parts:

> **Dendrites,** branches that receive input from other neurons,
>
> **Cell body,** which sustains the life of the cell and contains its DNA,
>
> **Axon,** a living cable that carries electrical impulses at very high speeds toward the dendrites of neighboring neurons.

A *synapse* is a junction between the axon of one neuron and the dendrite of another (or it can be between a neuron and a muscle). A synapse sends electrical or chemical (such as neurotransmitter) signals, which either excite or inhibit the chance for action. Each connection creates a weak electromagnetic field that can join together with the electromagnetic fields of other neural connections. Those combined connections increase the speed, empathy, and activity between neurons that are not in direct contact.[5]

The *glia,* or support cells for your neurons, are part of this electromagnetic "telepathy" of the brain. *Glial cells* are far more numerous than neurons, making up 90% of your brain's cells. They consume

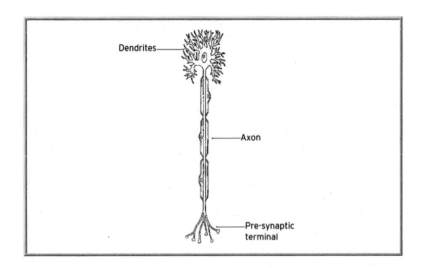

Dendrites

Axon

Pre-synaptic
terminal

parts of dead neurons, manufacture myelin (a white neuron coating
that protects the axon and increases axon impulses up to fifty times[6]),
form an immune system,[7] provide physical and nutritional support
for neurons, and even communicate with other synapses.[8]

Science is learning more about glial cells, adding to knowledge about neurons. Half of glial cells are tiny *granule cells,* which
hang out in the *cerebellum.* While the cerebellum (remember it's the
"little brain" of dough squeezed out the back of your wrist) makes
up only about 10% of the brain, it contains more nerve cells than
all the rest of the brain combined and is one of the brain's most
rapidly acting mechanisms.[9] It connects to the highest level of the
brain, the cerebral cortex, via 40 million nerve fibers. Compare
that to your optic track, which uses just 1 million to take care of
seeing and reading.

The *cerebral cortex* is our gray matter, composing about 85% of the
brain; it contains the lobes (frontal, parietal, temporal, and occipital).
The densely packed neurons in the cerebral cortex work together to
create *neural networks,* pathways of learning that constantly communicate and change.[10]

Are There Limits on Neurons?

There are two conflicting stories about our neurons: (1) we shouldn't kill our brain cells because they're the only ones we've got, and (2) neurogenesis—the birth of neurons—continues throughout our lives. What's the scoop?

Until the 1960s, scientists believed that whatever neurons we had at birth were all we'd get. But about that time, experiments on rats and monkeys showed otherwise; and still other experiments on canaries showed that they developed new brain cells when they learned new songs. Researchers wanted to know if people also developed new neurons—but since it's a little tricky to dissect the brain of a learning human, they couldn't find out that way for sure.

Move ahead thirty years to the '90s, when scientists conducted research on terminal cancer patients who were given certain drugs labeled with fluorescent dyes in their medical treatment. After the patients died, their brains were examined. The examinations showed that the patients had generated new neurons—right up until death. They indicated that the human hippocampus, a memory center of the limbic system, retains its ability to generate neurons throughout life.[11]

The Myth of Limited Brain Use

Is it true that we use only 10% of our brain? Do we have 90% that's just twiddling its proverbial thumbs, wishing it had something to do already? Does that idle 90% mean we are really psychic or could move mountains if we used it?

No, that's a myth, says neuroscientist Eric Chudler, director of education and outreach at the University of Washington and developer of the informative *Neuroscience for Kids* website.[12] Images from PET scans and MRI have shown that if someone loses 90% of her brain—or of any part of her brain—she will not just continue living as if nothing had happened. From the perspective of evolution, it does not make a whole lot of sense to build and maintain a massively underutilized organ.

Researchers still have questions about neurogenesis. New neurons in rat brains travel from the hippocampus to other parts of the brain, but researchers have not yet proven whether the same thing happens in human brains. Some camps question whether the new brain cells are neurons or glial cells and what purpose they serve.[13]

For us nonscientists, the important thing to know is that even though we get almost all our neurons at birth, our brains continue to change and grow, supporting our learning with new neurons, new connections, or both.

Connecting the Neurons

More important than how many main cells we have is how we use and connect the ones that stick around. These connections create maps (neural pathways) that constantly change as our moldable brain grows, learns, and matures. Those brain circuits that we actively maintain will remain and even grow stronger.

Your neural pathways constantly change as your brain grows, learns, and matures.

Researchers at Virginia University found that abilities based on accumulated knowledge keep increasing until age sixty.[14] However, this study's results were based on behavior, not the biology of the brain; it also does not address the effects of practice on strengthening cognition.[15]

When you take up a new hobby, like playing the guitar or knitting, your brain designates more cell power to this new activity. As you stick with it, the brain accommodates this new knowledge by changing or creating neural maps and maybe even assigning extra neurons to help. You go from remembering what fingers to use for the C-minor chord to just knowing it. What if you stop for a while? If you're a winter knitter, don't worry—those neural connections won't disappear over the summer. They just focus on something else. They'll be there next winter, though it might take them a little time to get their knit-purl connections back.

Practice may not always make perfect, but it does help you rearrange your neurons and connections. Don't worry about feeling dumb while you're learning. You're just ushering your neurons into place.

Is Your Brain a Boy or a Girl?

Here's a stunning revelation: men and women are different. But what differences are the results of nature (the brain and biology) and what differences are the results of nurture (parenting and culture)? Male and female brains have been compared for over a century, but the excitement really heated up in the past decade, as new tools have measured brain activity, sizes of brain areas, and behavioral responses.

News about the differences between men's and women's brains popped up everywhere—from John Gray's *Men Are from Mars, Women Are from Venus* and Louann Brizendine's *The Female Brain* to Discovery Health and *Newsweek*. All of these sources said that brain differences, present from birth, are what make men and women distinct. Even a former president of Harvard said that, based on brain research, women didn't have the brains for math and physics.[16]

These new discoveries were accepted by the media and public, but they were publicized without rigorous analysis. Recent scrutiny questions the validity of the studies and the hidden assumptions beneath the results.

Brain Sex Rumors

New studies of brains use functional magnetic resonance imaging (fMRI) and positron emission tomography (PET), both of which measure blood flow and produce three-dimensional imaging. Researchers compared male and female brains and compared the brains of those doing puzzles to those meditating, those looking at happy pictures or at sad ones, or those just listening or responding actively in a conversation. They've measured the sizes of brain components and the blood flow to areas that were active; the results were pictures of brains filled with bright blobs of color indicating which sections were active.

These studies aimed to show that male and female brains are significantly different at birth in many areas. Supposedly:

- Males have better right-hemisphere skills, such as those involved in art, music, and math, due to the testosterone male embryos receive; females are better at communicating, observing, and processing emotion.

- Males are better able to systematize and are more aggressive than females, also because of this infusion of testosterone in male embryos; females have more collaborative and verbal brains.

- Compared to men, women have the stronger ability to "mirror" others, feeling what others are feeling or sensing what others are thinking.

- Men have a larger amygdala, dubbed the "instinctual core of the brain," than women.

- Women worry more than men because their anterior cingulate cortex is larger.

- Women have more neurons for language processing and comprehension in the temporal lobe cortex than men have.

- The corpus callosum, a pathway of 200 to 250 million nerve fibers between the right and left hemispheres, is larger in women than in men. This greater number of cross-brain connections means women are better at activities involving both sides of the brain, and men are better at activities requiring the focus of one side or the other.

But several authors have called these studies on the carpet. They scientifically challenged whether (1) our advanced instruments tell as much as we'd like, (2) the assumptions they tell are true, and (3) the studies are large enough for their statistics to have veracity.

For instance, when looking at the corpus callosum, some studies found that it is the same size in men and women, and other studies found that it's bigger in men. Studies also question whether having a larger right hemisphere means increased learning or more difficulty learning. And while the anterior cingulate cortex is the part of the brain that generates worry, this part is also involved with a wide variety of cognitive, motor, and emotional tasks, such as decision-making;

so it makes as much sense to say that a larger anterior cingulate cortex means women think better than men, instead of that women worry more.

Cordelia Fine, author of *Delusions of Gender*, says that these studies are looking at the brain through traditional assumptions. It's just like 1915, she says, when studies "proved" that women couldn't judge political initiatives and couldn't vote, all because they had smaller upper spinal cords. The results of these studies are similarly biased because of what she calls *neurosexism.* [17]

We are starting to get larger and more valid studies about gender and the brain, which we hope will clarify the issue. And we know some consistent male-female brain differences in animals and humans from previous decades of study.

What Do We Really Know?

Boys and girls' brains are different at birth, but the differences are much smaller than we think, says Lise Eliot, PhD, in *Pink Brain, Blue Brain: How Small Differences Grow Into Troublesome Gaps—And What We Can Do About It.*[18]

In fact, before the eighth week of pregnancy, there is no male brain at all—everyone starts as a female. Around the eighth week, male embryos (meaning embryos with XY chromosomes) get a surge of testosterone. The testosterone changes the brain's original plan to create a uterus and ovaries in the female with XX chromosomes; the male embryo develops a penis and testicles instead.

Only a few physical pre-adolescent brain differences have been reliably proven to exist:

- Boys' brains are larger than girls' brains. (This difference used to support the idea that men were smarter, but when you consider the brains of elephants, the logic fades. Larger brains are needed for larger muscles and to process more sensations.[19])

- Girls' brains finish growing about one to two years earlier than boys' brains. (Hormonal differences are key in this growth difference.)

Brain Fitness for Women

- Parts of the *hypothalamus* are different. The hypothalamus controls basic body cycles and is connected to the pituitary (or "master hormone") gland. The areas of the hypothalamus that are different in males and females control circadian rhythms and reproduction.

There may be some subtle differences in boys and girls' sensory processing, language circuits, and frontal-lobe development, but overall, boys' brains and girls' brains are remarkably similar.

So what creates more gender-typical behavior? How babies are treated, say both Eliot and Fine. Our wonderfully plastic brains respond to gender-specific atmospheres. For example, if you believe you're better at math, the area of your brain that does math work will be larger. Even intentionally unbiased child-rearing practices have some sex stereotyping, according to Fine. Add Disney movies and sports stars to the mix, and it's a challenge to separate and study the natural brain from the nurtured one.

Hormones, such as testosterone, estradiol, oxytocin, and thyroid hormone, also affect both men and women's brains, causing differences in everything from pain response to aggression and emotional responses. In the next chapter, we'll talk about how the range of hormones affects functions of the brain.

Despite the popularity of studies that say sex differences are hardwired into brain structures, right now that assertion appears to be unproven. We have so much to learn about whether and how much gender behavior is influenced by differences in brains and hormones —even the best neuroscientists are still learning.

So when you're sorting through all the latest studies mentioned on Google News or articles in *Newsweek,* withhold your wholehearted approval until you've seen multiple large-sample studies. Some research might say you were born with limitations due to your gender, but others say that's not true. If you have to choose between thinking, "Oh well, that's just the kind of person I am," or thinking "I can move beyond my limitations and perceptions," why not go for the second?

No matter what your brain holds right now, from genetics to cultural reactions to annoying habits you learned from your parents, it has the ability to change. You can get a doctorate in diffusive biomolecular reactions, teach yourself to compartmentalize your emotional reactions, and learn the latest features on new cars—if you want.

---

*No matter what your brain holds right now,
it has the ability to change.*

No matter how you use your 125 trillion synapses, choose the path that gives you all the options you want. Then your brain will know it's working for a powerful and aware woman.

Chapter 3

Swimming in Different Hormones
Variations Beyond Brain Structure

On the one hand, [men will] never experience childbirth.
On the other hand, we can open all our own jars.

Bruce Willis, actor

When women are depressed, they eat or go shopping. Men invade
another country. It's a whole different way of thinking.

Elayne Boosler, comedian

Have you ever worked on those find-the-difference photo puzzles?
On one side, you see a picture of a celebrity like Beyoncé getting out
of her limo. Next to it is the same picture, but with a few changes: the
rearview mirror may be backwards, a fan in the background is missing, or there's an extra gold button on her jacket.

Male and female brains are kind of like those side-by-side pictures—mostly the same at birth but with a few differences.

Now imagine that the left picture of Beyoncé was swished in blue
tint and the right one in red. The pictures look different right away,
even before you look for the changed details.

Think of those colors as hormones. Hormones "tint" the parts of
the brain, changing some behavior, emotional responses, and even
vulnerability to illnesses. Certain parts of the brain readily absorb the
color and other parts don't.

Is everything colored by hormones? Yes and no. No matter how
much men and women differ from each other, the individual varia-
tions within the same sex are much wider. So while men as a group

tend to be more aggressive than women, you'll find *extremely* aggressive women and *extremely* timid men.

"Gender roles are flexible, reversible, and not all-or-none," says Donald Pfaff, PhD, author of *Man and Woman: An Inside Story*. "[B]iological influences on sex differences in brain and behavior operate at so many different levels, and they interact with environmental influences in so many different ways, that rigid, stereotyped ideas about what is and is not typical male or typical female behavior have become impossible to sustain."[20]

When you understand that you're swimming in different hormonal waters than men, you can have more compassion for yourself. You'll be open to the value of your brain's perspective on the world and be more relaxed with how wide the range of women's behaviors can be.

This chapter looks at hormones, both sexual and nonsexual, as well as other differences between men and women, including different responses and susceptibility to pain and illnesses.

Hormones

Hormones are chemicals released into the blood to activate or regulate bodily functions such as digestion, hunger, stress control, metabolism, growth, lactation, sex drive, circadian rhythm, and reproduction. Most hormones are secreted by specialized glands, like the thyroid gland in the throat, the pituitary gland in the brain, or the pancreas in the upper abdomen.

What's the difference between hormones and neurotransmitters? Hormones travel throughout the body via the bloodstream. Neurotransmitters, which activate and regulate such things as memory, learning, mood, behavior, sleep, pain perception, and sexual urges, travel across synapses in the neurons that make up the brain and nervous system. (Familiar neurotransmitters include serotonin, dopamine, and norepinephrine.)

Scientists have recently realized that in addition to hormones and neurotransmitters, we have neurohormones, which are hormones secreted by or acting on the nervous system.

Hormones are specialized for a wide array of functions, any of which can affect our brains.

Sexual Hormones

There are three basic sexual hormones: *androgens* (which are mainly male and include testosterone) and *estrogen* and *progesterone* (which are mainly female). Both men and women have all three types, but in different amounts, at different levels, and with different *receptors* (neurons specialized to be sensitive to certain chemicals, including hormones).

Oddly enough, testosterone can turn into estradiol, a type of estrogen. But no matter how complex they are or how they work, sexual hormones make sure that our bodies focus on mating and reproduction that species need to survive. And that can include behaviors that make boys be boys and girls be girls.

Many scientists are studying hormones and behavior in hopes of finding links between the two. For example, studies of the male population show that violent behavior peaks when men have increased testosterone, in the late teens and early twenties. But that doesn't necessarily mean that other behaviors often seen as gender specific are driven by sexual hormones. In other words, it isn't estrogen that makes some people put on makeup, have in-depth discussions about feelings, and shop until they drop, or testosterone that makes others leave their socks on the floor or become fascinated with construction.

The farther away from "nitty-gritty reproductive biology" we get, says Pfaff, the harder it is to clearly link the behavior with sexual hormones.[21] That's because the human brain is also influenced by so many things, including environment, childhood development, prenatal development, nutrition, toxins, hormones, the conscious mind, and the brain's own structure.

To further complicate things, sexual hormones are released not only as part of *internal* bodily functions, but also as a response to *external* experiences. Say you have a date with your spouse that includes dinner, a romantic movie, sweet talk, a candlelit bedroom, and soft fingertips caressing your belly. These external actions can get your estrogen going. Similarly, sexual drive, aggression, and social dominance can make testosterone rise in men. Many studies show a correlation—a coordinated relationship—between testosterone and certain behavior, but it's mostly not known if testosterone causes the behavior or vice versa.

The body can produce hormones in response to external experiences, such as a romantic evening.

"When you examine testosterone levels when males [in a study] are first placed together in a social group," said Robert Sapolsky, expert on testosterone from Stanford University, "testosterone levels predict nothing about who is going to be aggressive. Behavior drives the hormonal changes, rather than the other way around."[22]

So what are these primary sexual hormones that make things so complex?

Testosterone: Testosterone, the primary male hormone, has been shown to boost muscle mass and status-seeking/social-dominance behavior.[23] But the testosterone-fueled goal of getting to the top of the heap doesn't always lead to increased aggression; it could generate behaviors such as cooperating with others, if that helps men avoid rejection and, as a result, maintain their social standing.[24]

Testosterone is produced in the testicles of men, the ovaries of women, and in the adrenal glands of both sexes. In women, testosterone and other androgens can trigger responses similar to those of men, including increased muscle mass and social-dominance behaviors, and it is linked to sex drive. More is being learned about the role of androgens in women, but most scientific attention has been paid to estrogen and progesterone.

Estrogen: Estrogen, the primary female sex hormone, is produced by the ovaries and in small amounts by the liver, breasts, brain, and adrenal glands.[25] It has profound effects on just about every part of women's bodies: heart, bones, blood vessels, skin, hair, breasts, mucous membranes, pelvic muscles, and urinary and reproductive tracts.[26]

In the brain, estrogen affects attention, motor control, pain reception, mood, and memory. In women, estrogen helps regulate the brain's ability to learn and encode memories; testosterone may perform the same function in men, although as mentioned earlier, testosterone makes estrogen.[27]

Women experience greater fluctuations of estrogen, which can affect women's moods, stress, and learning.[28] Low estrogen may increase depression and compulsive behaviors. That's because estrogen regulates emotion in several ways, including:

- Increasing serotonin and serotonin receptors, which regulate mood, sleep, and learning,
- Modifying the production and effects of endorphins, the "feel-good" neurotransmitter,
- Protecting nerves from damage and perhaps stimulating nerve growth.[29]

Progesterone: This hormone is involved in pregnancy, regulating everything from sex drive, ovulation, the uterine lining, maintenance of pregnancy, and lactation—in short, everything you'd want and need to have a baby.

Much of what we understand about progesterone's effects comes from what happens to our bodies when it's low: infertility, insomnia, sore breasts, weight gain, water retention, vaginal dryness, and decreased sex drive.[30] Lowered levels can even cause migraine headaches, depression, panic attacks, abnormal menstrual cycles, and blood-sugar problems.[31]

Beyond its role as the pregnancy hormone, progesterone has neuro-protective properties and helps with traumatic brain injury by reducing swelling.[32] It is positively associated with increased social connection as well.[33]

Other Hormones

Even the amounts of certain nonsexual hormones (people have over fifty hormones) are different in men and women. What's also different is how sensitive each sex is to them and the disorders each sex can experience because of them. Here's look at three of these hormones.

Oxytocin: When you fall in love, want to cuddle, or are a mom of a baby and want to nurse, oxytocin is at work. Oxytocin (not *Oxycontin,* the prescribed painkiller) has major roles in

- Birth, lactation (releasing breast milk), and maternal bonding;
- Managing the circadian rhythm—your internal twenty-four-hour clock that determines when you want to fall asleep and wake up;[34]
- Trust and bonding via actions such as parenting, hugging, touching, and having orgasms—which is why it's called the "love hormone."[35]

Because women can give birth, we have more oxytocin than men, and it works better for us. Oxytocin is amplified by estrogen and counteracted by testosterone, says Marianne J. Legato, MD, FACP, author of *Why Men Never Remember and Women Never Forget* and founder of Columbia's Partnership for Gender-Specific Medicine.[36] That means that after sex, when you and your male partner both have a burst of loving oxytocin, you both want to cuddle and connect—at first. But testosterone counteracts the oxytocin, and the fact your sweetie might want to soon do something different, like check his e-mail, could have nothing to do with you.

Oxytocin has been used to induce labor, but more recently has been put into a nasal spray and marketed to helping with everything from autism and shyness to getting your man to share more in a relationship.[37]

Thyroid Hormone: The thyroid gland secretes a hormone that regulates metabolism, or how the body uses energy. Thyroid hormone affects a long list of items, including weight, body temperature, breathing, muscle strength, skin dryness, menstrual cycles, brain development, cholesterol levels, and heart and nervous-system functions. Just about every organ in your body can be affected by this one-ounce gland, shaped like a butterfly, that's located in the lower part of your neck.

Because of pregnancy, aging, and autoimmune disease, women's thyroids often get out of sync, sometimes producing too much thyroid hormone and, more often, too little. It can be hard to distinguish symptoms of thyroid problems from other concerns—such as depression, menopause, and fibromyalgia—and thyroid issues can make these concerns worse.

If you are *hyper*thyroid, with too much thyroid hormone, you may have some of these signs and symptoms:

- Nervousness, anxiety, irritability, and/or panic disorder;
- Increased perspiration and/or heat intolerance;
- Racing heart and palpitations (irregular heartbeats);
- Thinning skin and/or hair;
- Muscular weakness, especially in the upper arms and thighs;
- Shaky hands;
- Staring gaze;
- Insomnia and/or fatigue;
- More frequent bowel movements;
- Weight loss despite a good appetite;
- Lighter menstrual flow and/or less frequent menstrual periods.

Hyperthyroidism and one of its causes, Graves' disease (an autoimmune thyroid illness[38]), affect eight times as many women than men. Treatment depends on the cause of the hyperthyroidism and ranges from no treatment to antithyroid medication to radioactive iodine.

If you are *hypo*thyroid, with too little thyroid hormone, you may have these signs and symptoms:

- Fatigue, from feeling run down to exhaustion;
- Difficulty concentrating, brain fog;
- Depression, anxiety, and/or difficulty sleeping;
- Unexplained or excessive weight gain and appetite change;
- Dry, coarse, and/or itchy skin;

- Dry, coarse, and/or thinning hair;
- Feeling cold, especially in the extremities;
- Constipation;
- Heart palpitations;
- Muscle and joint pain;
- Infertility and/or miscarriages;
- Increased menstrual flow and more frequent periods.[39]

Like Graves' disease, Hashimoto's thyroiditis, an autoimmune disease that causes hypothyroidism, is also more common in women than in men; it affects roughly seven women for every one man.[40] Thyroid-hormone-replacement drugs are used for treatment of hypothyroidism. Many women who have suffered from thyroid problems notice a huge difference in their symptoms when they've recovered from thyroid-hormone imbalance.

Estrogen and other hormones can interact with thyroid hormone, making women more susceptible to thyroid problems—especially hypothyroidism—during and after pregnancy and during menopause.[41]

Pregnant moms need to have enough thyroid during pregnancy, especially during the first ten to twelve weeks, to help the baby's brain development, says endocrinologist Dr. Gunjan Tykodi.[42]

Melatonin: You may have heard of melatonin if you have sleep problems, because this hormone maintains the body's circadian rhythm, and regulates sleepiness, wakefulness, and body temperature. But melatonin has other critical functions. This hormone, secreted by the pineal gland in the middle of your head, also helps regulate other hormones and determines when teen girls start to menstruate, the frequency and duration of menstrual cycles, and the timing of menopause.

It also has strong antioxidant effects and may strengthen the immune system. Some think melatonin levels may be associated with breast-cancer risk, since women with breast cancer tend to have lower levels of melatonin.

What do you get your melatonin from? Darkness. Your pineal gland pumps out more melatonin when it's dark and stops producing the hormone when it's light. If you turn on the bathroom light in the middle of the night, you prompt your pineal to produce less melatonin, which is why you could have a harder time falling back asleep when you return to bed. Exposure to bright lights in the evening (when you work on the computer or watch TV late at night) or too little light during the day (when you're doing shift work or have jet lag) can disrupt the body's normal melatonin cycles. You might try software programs such as Flux and color filters to make computer screens more night friendly.[43]

Researchers believe melatonin levels drop as we age, which could be why some older adults have sleep problems. This change in levels could be why older adults tend to go to bed and wake up early.[44]

To increase your nightly melatonin, start with a melatonin-friendly lifestyle: use dusk and dawn as reminders to go to bed and wake up, make sure the bedroom is dark, and keep a dim light in the bathroom at night.

Melatonin supplements—tablets, capsules, cream, and lozenges that dissolve under the tongue—may help with sleep problems associated with menopause. Check with your doctor, and keep the dose close to the amount that our bodies normally produce (less than 0.3 mg per day).[45]

Men, Women, and Illness

Women get sick more often than men. A survey of 3,000 people, conducted by Engage Mutual, a British insurance and financial company, found that women get sick an average of seven times a year and men an average of five times.[46] There can be many reasons—stress, greater exposure to toxins, the vulnerability of pregnancy. But a key piece, especially in susceptibility to autoimmune illnesses, is sexual hormones.

"It's pretty difficult to find any single factor that's more predictive for [certain] diseases than gender," said Thomas Insel, the head of the National Institute of Mental Health.[47]

While more men than women experience extreme aggression, autism spectrum disorders, Gulf War Syndrome, and adult attention deficit hyperactivity disorder (ADHD), women are more likely than men to suffer from the following health problems, which can add to stress on the brain.

Autoimmune Illnesses

About 75% of all autoimmune disorders happen in women.[48] In auto-immune syndromes, such as fibromyalgia, chronic fatigue immune dysfunction syndrome (CFIDS), lupus, Hashimoto's in the thyroid, multiple chemical sensitivity, and rheumatoid arthritis.[49] A patient's immune or infection-protecting defenses turn back against her and attack some of her own healthy functional cells and tissues.[50]

"Sex hormones influence the onset and severity of immune . . . conditions," says an article in the *American Journal of Pathology.*[51] That's partly because immune cells have receptors for estrogen and andro-gens (e.g., testosterone). While androgens and perhaps progestogens may protect from autoimmune disease, says the *Oxford Journal of Rheumatology,*[52] estrogen mostly stimulates the immune system.[53]

Insomnia

Over 60% of insomnia sufferers are women. Women are susceptible to the common insomnia causes, such as stress, irregular sleep hours, certain foods, caffeine, smoking, lack of exercise, and too much light, often from computers and TV.

But insomnia is also affected by hormonal fluctuations. That means you may wake at night or struggle to fall asleep on premenstrual nights, during perimenopause, and after menopause.[54] The common tribulations of motherhood, such as being nine months pregnant, having a baby who wants to nurse, or having a young child who wants to sleep with you, certainly make sleeping a challenge.

To learn how to relax and sleep well at night, check out chapter 5.

Depression

Women who suffer from chronic anxiety and stress are more likely to get depressed. Everyday stress is one thing, but women who have had childhood or other trauma (an estimated 20% of women[55]) are more likely than other women to experience depression. The ratio of females to males who have depression is 2.5 to 1 in the United States.

Depression and its symptoms—lack of initiation, loss of pleasure, disrupted daily circadian rhythms, anxiety, sleep disturbances—dampen the arousal pathways in the brain. Fortunately, exercise, talk therapy, and the right medicine can help reawaken the brain to new paths instead of just depression.

Seasonal Affective Disorder (SAD)

Seasonal affective disorder can range from winter blues to depression. Over 75% if those who have it are women, and the majority of them are in their twenties to thirties.[56]

What causes SAD? There are several hypotheses:

- Oversecretion of melatonin in the winter,
- Lack of light, which stimulates specialized cells in the retina that directly connect the eyes to the brain,[57]
- Body-chemistry problems causing the neurotransmitters dopamine and serotonin to be out of sync and thus interfere with mood, appetite, and sleep patterns,[58]
- Lack of vitamin D.

If you can't move to Costa Rica from November to March, light boxes can help SAD. Check with your doctor about increasing your vitamin D as well.

Anorexia Nervosa

Women who experience anorexia nervosa may have a hypersensitivity to estrogen in the hypothalamus. That part of the brain produces hormones to control body temperature, hunger, moods, and the release of hormones from different glands. This hypersensitivity may create the sensation of having eaten enough before the body is full.

Migraines

A migraine is more than a headache. It's a neurological disease that can include nausea and vomiting; sensitivity to light, touch, and sound;

tingling or other sensations in the skin; visual changes, like seeing an aura, halo, or zigzag of lights; sound auras, such as echoes, tremolo, or buzzing; hunger pangs; and slurred speech. And some people get migraines without even the headache.

Not fun, as anyone who's ever had a migraine knows. About one out of twenty men and one out of five women get migraines— chronically (more than half the days each month), periodically (perhaps with the menstrual cycle) and/or episodically (not predictably).

Boys get more migraines than girls—until they reach puberty. Migraines become a predominantly female issue after menstruation begins; women are twice as likely to have migraines around their period, and migraines can be most severe during menstruation. But it's the fluctuation of hormones that can set off migraine sensitivity. For many women with migraines, natural menopause is a blessing, because the hormonal fluctuation ceases.

In addition to hormones, other things, such as food, lights, and red wine, can trigger migraines. But the triggers aren't the cause of migraines. The brain's hypersensitivity is the cause, says Carolyn Bernstein, MD, in her book *The Migraine Brain*.[59] A hypersensitive brain reacts frequently and intensely to brain stress by creating an electrical wave, a red alert, that can make the nervous system go haywire. The electrical-wave reaction isn't unusual, but the over-responsiveness of the migraine brain is.

The effects of the wave can start with physical sensitivity—clothes suddenly feel tight, the head feels hot. Then the wave can incite pain in one or both of the major nerves that run on either side of the head, from behind the ear to the forehead, nose, and jaw. That is why one side of the head may hurt and one of the eyes can throb.

The migraine brain even looks different than a regular brain when seen through a brain scan. Scans done at Massachusetts General Hospital showed that the part of the brain that processes pain, touch, temperature, and sensory information—the somatosensory cortex—was 21% thicker than the somatosensory cortices of those who don't experience migraines.[60] That thinner somatosensory cortex either causes the migraines or is the result of them—researchers don't know yet.

Those affected often are vigilant about avoiding what sets them off. That can mean getting sufficient sleep and avoiding low blood sugar, alcohol and/or red wine, the artificial sweetener aspartame, foods containing the amino acid tryanine (such as soy sauce, pepperoni, bananas, and raspberries), toxic cleaning fluids and chemicals, smoke, strong smells, and computers or video games.

Some migraine sufferers are helped by over-the-counter drugs, including those with caffeine. Others use the medication Imitrex, part of the triptan family, which interrupts the biomechanical pain/brain-wave effect. Many get some help from magnesium supplements, since those with migraines have lower levels of this mineral. Interestingly, tinted glasses can also help stabilize brain activity, says a study from Michigan State University and the University of Michigan.[61]

Stress

Is life harder for women than it is for men? Whether it is or not, women have more intense responses to stress and anxiety disorders, says Margaret Altemus of Cornell University Medical School.[62] The reasons are women's hormone reactions and the way the neurons operate in women's brains:

- We release greater amounts of cortisol (stress hormone) from the adrenal glands.

- Our brains trigger greater physical responses in the automatic nervous system, such as breathing changes, increased heart rate, stomach tension, and sweating.

- Estrogen increases production of corticotropin-releasing factor (CRF), a brain protein that tells the pituitary gland to send out stress messages to the adrenal glands.

You'll learn what stress does to your body and brain, and how to handle it, in chapter 5.

Pain

Being a woman is a pain—and that's not just an expression.

Researchers at Florida State University combined the statistics from over eighty different pain disorders and found that, compared to men, twice as many women suffered from pain disorders. "The burden of pain is greater, more varied and variable for women than men," says pain expert Karen Berkley, PhD, distinguished research professor of neuroscience at Florida State.[63] One reason that women have more pain is unsurprising: disorders of the uterus can radiate pain.

Another reason is that women's XX chromosomes "lead to a fair number of painful diseases that men simply would not get," says Donald Pfaff, PhD, author of *Man and Woman: An Inside Story.*[64]

A third reason for more pain in women is surprising: women are more likely than men to have low blood pressure (59% of women have low pressure versus 43% of men), according to British physicians' research.[65] In general, the lower the pressure, the greater the sensitivity to pain.

Men and women's brains also receive and act on pain signals differently. It's a complex story of neurons and receptors, but here's the simple version: there are neurons that cause partial amnesia to moderate pain, and males have more receptors for these neurons.

And then there is how hormones affect pain. The good news is that during childbirth, estrogen and progesterone combine to stimulate opiumlike particles and receptors on the spinal cord and significantly reduce a woman's perception of pain.[66] The bad news is that in ordinary life, estrogen has different receptors. Some decrease and some increase pain, and they are all scattered throughout the nervous system.

Women are not whiny wimps when it comes to pain. Men just have more resources in their brains to help them "suck it up" and ignore pain.

Are We More Than Our Hormones?

We're swimming in a sea of hormones, and they have some strong currents. Because of hormones, your baby clock might start to tick as you approach age thirty. You might snap at your husband, then sincerely apologize the next day when you get your period. You could cringe at even the thought of a migraine, or you might have to deal with a weird autoimmune disease that destroys your blood platelets.

Still, hormones are not all you are. You have choices when it comes to dealing with the ebb and flow of hormonal currents, such as learning to be content with or without children, finding a different way to express your emotions, feeling joyful when you wake headache free, and managing your autoimmune disease with diet or medicine.

And underneath these choices, you know that you are more than your illnesses, children, and emotions. That's not often easy to remember in daily life, but knowing you're more than what happens and how you feel allows you to step back, relax into the life you have, and experience a changed perspective on the flow of all that estrogen, progesterone, oxytocin, and whatever else is dancing in your brain and body.

Keep reading to learn more about what that dance is like for women, and some choices that may make life easier.

Chapter 4

The Brain During
Menstruation and Menopause

*If men could menstruate, clearly, menstruation would become an envi-
able, boast-worthy, masculine event: Men would brag about how long
and how much. Sanitary supplies would be federally funded and free.
Of course, some men would still pay for the prestige of such commercial
brands as Paul Newman Tampons, Muhammad Ali's Rope-a-Dope
Pads, John Wayne Maxi Pads, and Joe Namath Jock Shields—"For
Those Light Bachelor Days."*

Gloria Steinem, feminist, journalist, and activist

*There is no more creative force in the world
than the menopausal woman with zest.*

Margaret Mead, pioneering anthropologist

When Sherree read about menopause or hormone supplements,
she became anxious. Everything seemed to say that (1) menopause
was hell, (2) life without estrogen was barely manageable, and (3)
hormone-replacement pills increased the risk of developing breast
cancer, heart disease, blood clotting, and dementia.[67]

Still, her female coworkers in their late fifties seemed fine. She
overheard some of them saying that they weren't on hormone replacement therapy (HRT, they called it), though one of them said she had
less brain fog and felt much saner and happier when she began HRT.

Sherree, age forty-four, wished she knew what was in store for her.
She didn't know if her mom had had an easy or rough menopause,

since she had died right after Sherree got her first period, at age twelve. And even if Sherree did know about her mother, would menopause would be the same for her as it was for her mom?

Science always has more to learn, but there are some things we do know about hormones, our bodies, and our brains—how they work monthly and throughout our lives.

Estrogen, the Wonder Hormone

Sherree had always been told that estrogen was the female plague, making her moody, bloated, and covered with zits every month. Actually, it wasn't estrogen that caused these discomforts, but the fluctuations of hormones and how they balanced with each other—or didn't.[68]

Still, estrogen itself is quite a phenomenon. It plays a large role in directing our entire nervous system, which can affect the heart, stomach, liver, pancreas, and immune system. Our brains can operate without estrogen, but not as well as they do with it. Think of estrogen in the brain like toothpaste when you brush your teeth—makes them cleaner than just the toothbrush itself.

Estrogen multiplies the synapses between neurons,[69] keeps synapses flexible, and supports the growth of dendrites (the twigs on the synapse tree that conduct electrochemical stimulation).[70] That helps when you learn a new language or how to do a handstand in yoga.

Estrogen assists the dopamine neurons, helping stabilize brain activity, regulate the flow of information between parts of the brain, and control movement and balance, as well as making you feel happy. It also protects your neurons from degenerative diseases, like Parkinson's.[71]

The problem appears when our natural wonder drug leaves town to become a star in Hollywood. To understand what happens to our brains then, let's flash back to when estrogen was an ingénue.

Hormones on Center Stage for Puberty

Three hormones start the dance of a girl's body into womanhood. Sometime between ages ten and fourteen, the brain triggers a release of *luteinizing hormone* (LH) and *follicle-stimulating hormone* (FSH) from the pituitary gland. These two hormones stimulate estrogen production in the ovaries. (In boys, LH and FSH stimulate testosterone and sperm production.)

The domino effect of hormonal changes includes a rise in dopamine and oxytocin (the "love hormone"). The neurotransmitter dopamine stimulates the brain's pleasure and motivation circuits.

Other hormones active in puberty are androgens, which are associated with aggression and sexual response. One type of androgen is testosterone, and another is dihydroepiandrosterone (DHEA). Androgens are primarily male hormones, though females also have them, and girls who have higher levels of DHEA and testosterone tend to have sex earlier than girls with lower levels. Ironically, a good countermeasure for these high levels is oral contraceptives.[72] They reduce sex drive and aggression because they suppress the androgens produced by ovaries.

Hormones and Aunt Flo (or Your Monthly Visitor)

In our teens, we begin making the monthly menstrual-hormone journey, a voyage of the body and the brain. You're familiar with the route:

It starts with the irritation and/or relief of your period ...

moves into the "just fine" weeks that follow ...

may encounter a cramp or ache during ovulation ...

then goes through the week or two that ranges from just fine to the hell of PMS, until you reach ...

the irritation and/or relief of your period.

Such is life for most women for forty years, starting in the preteen or early teen years.

Here's the map of what's happening within your body and brain during the trip.

In the follicular phase, before ovulation, your body pumps up follicles (cavities in the ovary containing the immature egg) with the aptly named follicle-stimulating hormone (FSH), and luteinizing hormone (LH). Both endorphin and estrogen levels are high, giving a real boost to neurotransmitters such as serotonin, dopamine, and norepinephrine. The result? You feel pretty good.

The follicles get all pumped and tell the ovary to release the egg, about fourteen days after the first day of the previous period. Estrogen rapidly spikes and drops during ovulation, and it seems to prime your sensitivity to the next drop in estrogen a few days before your period.[73]

The egg begins its journey down the fallopian tubes and begins the luteal phase, when the body prepares a home for a possible fertilized egg. During the first part of the luteal phase, the scar *(corpus luteum)* on the ovary where the egg used to live produces estrogen and progesterone to care for the egg, if it's fertilized.

Estrogen refreshes and recharges cells and areas of your brain, which helps you be more socially relaxed, sharper, and steadier on the emotional level. Progesterone helps the brain by boosting the receptors to enhance GABA (gamma-aminobutyric acid), a neurotransmitter that slows down or calms the nervous system in the brain, which can help reduce anxiety.

Premenstrual Haze

During the premenstrual days (the second part of your luteal phase) your corpus luteum scar realizes its egg is not going to be fertilized,[74] and it crumbles. It stops producing estrogen and progesterone, and your body gets ready to shed the uterine lining it had created just in case the sperm and egg had a shindig.

Your body and brain do not like the loss of estrogen and progesterone, nor do they like having more estrogen than progesterone.[75] Their reactions range from slight fatigue, tension, or emotional stress to more potent symptoms that keep you from functioning.

The drop in estrogen reduces the production of serotonin, the neurotransmitter that regulates mood, appetite, and sensory perception. Estrogen no longer recharges your brain, so you may feel not as sharp, socially adept, or emotionally steady. The drop of progesterone levels means the brain doesn't have nearly enough receptors for GABA, the soothing brain chemical.[76] So the GABA is essentially wasted.

To add fuel to the fire, women have more *prostaglandins* during this time. Prostaglandins are fatty acids that, on the good side, stimulate the contraction of smooth muscle and the uterus. On the not-so-good side, in the premenstrual week, they cause inflammation, sensitize the spinal nerves to pain, increase bloating, and congregate in the brain, breasts, and reproductive tract, making all three hurt.[77] Pain relievers such as Advil (ibuprofen), Aleve (naproxen), and Midol all help at this time because they are anti-inflammatory and/or prostaglandin blockers.

Your poor limbic (primitive) brain also goes into withdrawal. It no longer connects as well to the cerebral cortex, and you have less access to your skills for handling strong emotional reactions.

Your brain can also go "on strike" during these days. Bruce McEwen, renowned professor of neuroscience at Rockefeller University, says all these hormone shifts overload your brain's self-regulatory systems (called *allostatic loading)* and overcome your brain's capacity to compensate.[78]

Your brain also gets triggered to respond to more food cues, which may not be all bad.[79] Your brain might want you to consume chocolate, which has magnesium salts, a mineral that can help with depression.[82]

Premenstrual Syndrome, Dysphoria, Depression, and More

Premenstrual days mildly affect 75 to 80% of women, says the Women's Health Study.[81] Symptoms include irritability, crying, depression, oversensitivity, moods, insomnia, fatigue, bloating, change in sexual interest, headaches, backaches, cramps, aggression, nausea, joint pain, acne, dizziness, and confusion or a lack of concentration ability.

For most of us, the premenstrual week is only annoying. You may have to watch what you say, but your symptoms don't really impair your ability to function. The American College of Obstetricians and Gynecologists estimates at least 85% of menstruating women have at least one premenstrual syndrome (PMS) symptom, and the symptoms they experience are fairly mild and don't need treatment.[82] But 20 to 50% of women find that their symptoms interfere somewhat with daily activities, according to the University of Maryland Medical Center.[83] When these symptoms become so intense that women are unable to function (which happens to 3 to 8% of women), the diagnosis changes from PMS to premenstrual dysphoric disorder (PMDD).[84] (For simplicity, I'll generally refer to this monthly stress as PMS.)

You might feel all alone when you are in the depths of PMS. But while no one can infuse you with a shower of sunshine or keep your house perpetually clean, you have options. These treatments may reduce the intensity of PMS from that of a cyclone roller coaster to that of a drive on a bumpy road, or maybe even make it as smooth as a limousine ride. As always, check with your doctor before trying anything new, especially when changing or adding supplements or herbs or if your PMS continues to be a problem.

Prevention: What you do with your body during the weeks and months before your period can influence how your body handles the hormone roller coaster.

> **Move more.** Ideally, move until you sweat for thirty minutes and then do it again five days each week. But if you can't quite do that, keep steadily increasing your exercise. Women who exercise regularly are less likely to have symptoms of PMS, says the University of Maryland Medical Center.[85]

> **If you smoke, quit.** Women between the ages of twenty-seven and forty-four who smoke are twice as likely to develop PMS, according to a study published in the American Journal of Epidemiology.[86]

> **Try a low-fat diet.** Studies have linked higher dietary fat, especially diets high in saturated and trans fats, with higher prostaglandin levels, which cause PMS aches and pains.[87]

> **Become a vegetarian.** Women following a low-fat vegetarian diet significantly reduced menstrual pain and PMS symptoms, according to a study conducted by the Physicians Committee for Responsible Medicine with Georgetown University's Department of Obstetrics and Gynecology.[88]

Check out possible food allergens, including dairy, wheat (gluten), soy, corn, preservatives, and food additives.

Eat fewer red meats and more lean meats, cold-water fish, tofu (soy), or beans for protein.

Use healthy cooking oils, such as olive oil or vegetable oil.

During the Premenstrual Week: While the following are good things to do regularly, they can help even if you wait until the premenstrual week to do them.

- **Decrease your consumption of salt, caffeine, alcohol, artificial sweeteners, and sugar.** You don't have to suffer; just pick one thing to reduce or eliminate for a month or two to see if it makes a difference.

- **Stay hydrated.** Drink six to eight glasses of water a day and/or get some liquid from your fruits, veggies, and other foods. Water flushes toxins and can help reduce bloating.

- **Increase your calcium intake.** Eat calcium-rich foods, including beans, almonds, and dark green leafy vegetables, such as spinach and kale. Calcium-enriched soy milk helps with symptoms of PMS. (See more about supplements below.)

- **Move.** Yes, I'm repeating myself. Movement/exercise raises serotonin and balances dopamine and norepinephrine (all mood neurotransmitters). It stabilizes a broad range of variables, toning down the ripple effect of shifting hormones. Push through the inertia and get the payoffs from moving.

Medications: Your doctor or medical team may prescribe or suggest the following medications:

Diuretics for bloating and water retention.

Ibuprofen (Advil, Motrin) and **naproxen** (Aleve), which are nonsteroidal anti-inflammatory drugs (NSAIDs) that help with headaches, cramps, and levels of the inflammatory prostaglandins.

Antidepressants to relieve many mood symptoms, especially if your emotions overtake you. Working with a doctor experienced with these medicines can help you find the one that's right for you.

Birth control pills to stop ovulation and keep hormone levels stable.

Supplements: For the one or two of us who don't have perfect diets, these supplements can be helpful to our brains on PMS:[89]

Multivitamins. Choose one containing the antioxidant vitamins A, C, and E; the B-complex vitamins; and trace minerals, such as magnesium, calcium, zinc, and selenium.

Calcium. If you don't get enough in your diet, several studies suggest that taking 500 to 1,000 mg calcium citrate daily and 400 IU vitamin D daily. These may reduce PMS symptoms and are also good for your bones.

Magnesium. Take 400 mg daily. Magnesium is a calming mineral and a muscle relaxant, which makes it good for cramps. It may also reduce breast tenderness, bloating, migraines, and fluid retention. High doses of magnesium can lower blood pressure and may cause loose stools.[90] You can get some magnesium in greens, halibut, nuts such as almonds and cashews, sesame seeds, flax, and whole grains. And there's some in chocolate, too.

Omega-3 fatty acids, such as fish oils. One or two capsules daily of about 1,050 mg of EPA and 150 mg of DHA or one tablespoonful of oil helps reduce menstrual cramps (per University of Maryland Medical Center) and internal inflammation.[91] Omega-3s may also prevent or alleviate bloating and improve brain function, which contributes to mood balance and emotional health.[92] Talk to your doctor if you're taking any blood-thinning medication.

Herbs: Herbs have been used for millennia as natural medicines, which means they are medicines. They can interfere with other pharmaceutical medications and may have side effects. Let your doctor know what herbs you're thinking of taking and ask his or her opinion.

Herbs come in many formats including pills, teas, tinctures, and liquid extracts. Make sure you have a standardized extract with consistent potency in each dosage.

Chaste tree or chasteberry *(Vitex agnus castus)* may help reduce symptoms of PMS, including headache, irritability, and breast tenderness, say several studies. Take 400 mg daily before breakfast. It may interfere with medications, such as birth control pills, antipsychotics, and estrogen supplements. If you have a hormone-sensitive condition, such as endometriosis or breast cancer, check with your doctor before taking.

Dandelion *(Taraxacum officinale)* leaf tincture, 5 to 10 mL taken two or three times a day, will help with the fluid retention associated with PMS. You can also prepare teas from the leaf. Dandelion can interact with a number of medications, including lithium and some antibiotics, and can cause a reaction in persons allergic to ragweed.

Black cohosh *(Actaea racemosa),* 20 to 40 mg, two times a day, is sometimes suggested to reduce PMS symptoms, though scientific evidence doesn't consistently support its effects. Black cohosh may interact with a number of medications. If you have a history of hormone-related conditions or of liver or kidney disease, ask your doctor before taking black cohosh.

Evening primrose oil *(Oenothera biennis),* 500 to 1,000 mg daily, is a source of gamma linolenic acid (GLA); you can convert about 5% of it to the longer-chain omega-3 oils our brains need. It may increase the risk of bleeding. Although some clinical trials have shown a benefit of evening primrose oil for PMS, the best-designed trials found no effect.

St. John's wort *(Hypericum perforatum),* 300 mg taken two to three times per day may relieve the depression associated with PMS. St. John's wort interacts with a number of other medications and herbs, especially birth control pills. It must be taken consistently throughout the month for best results. Direct sun exposure may cause rashes in some people taking it.

Emotional Care: You can help with PMS by learning to respond differently to your emotional reactions, instead of just blasting those who bug the hell out of you.

> **Psychological acupressure.** Techniques such as the Emotional Freedom Technique (EFT) and Tapas Acupressure Technique (TAT) can help you release body tension and habitual patterns of emotions before you blow up. They're described in chapter 7.

> **Body care.** Use this time to be gentle and loving with your body, indulging in a longer bath, taking an extra yoga class, or getting someone to rub your back—try a little massage roller ball.

> **Get support for trauma.** Fifty to 60% of the women with PMDD may have sexual- or physical-abuse histories. That is much greater than the 20 to 25% expected of women in the general population. Your PMS may indicate that you could use support about something that happened a long while ago—something your body has not forgotten.

> **Grow as a person.** Even if your PMS is not from trauma, what sets you off is still likely a problem even during the ordinary days. Noticing what you react to can help you better understand yourself and make changes in how you experience your life.

Other Options:

> **Homeopathy.** It works best when a homeopath prescribes a remedy specific to subtle symptoms; however, few studies have examined homeopathy's effectiveness.

> **Acupuncture.** Some studies show that acupuncture can help with PMS.[93] Treatments may include moxibustion (the herb mugwort is heated over certain acupuncture points), herbal treatment, and/or changes to the diet.

> **Chiropractic.** Women with PMS have been found to have more back problems, physical tenderness, and muscle weakness. One study showed that PMS symptoms significantly decreased after women received

chiropractic spinal and soft-tissue therapy, though treatments may be needed monthly to maintain the results.

Do Alternative PMS Treatments Really Work?

Some alternative treatments for PMS have been shown to work in some studies, but not in others. However, studies may or may not reflect all there is to know about the effectiveness of an alternative treatment; for example, the dosage of an herb may not be right or may be affected if it's taken with or without food. Studies let you know how a population reacts; individuals may have success that is not reflected in the studies.

Some folks reject alternative treatments, saying these treatments work only because of the placebo effect: the notion that people feel better because they *believe* they're taking a useful medicine when they're actually taking a harmless medicine or procedure.

Harvard University and Beth Israel Deaconess Medical Center did a study where they told participants with irritable bowel syndrome (IBS) to take a placebo (a sugar pill) twice a day. The bottle even had "placebo" written on the label. Compared to the control group that took no medicine—real or pretend—the placebo group reported a significant relief from their IBS symptoms (59% compared to 35% of the control group). And get this: the rates of improvement experienced by those on the placebo were roughly equivalent to those taking the most powerful medicines for IBS.[94]

Does the placebo effect mean alternative treatments don't actually work? Maybe, maybe not. One of the most significant factors in health and life is how our body and mind work together. Be open to finding what can help you—regardless of how it does so—and you will have more opportunities for a healthier body and brain throughout your menstrual cycle.

When There's a Bun in the Oven:
Hormonal Changes During Pregnancy

If you get pregnant, hormones from both you and your baby have a field day (or more like field months). Because of these hormonal changes, along with strong emotions and adjustment to parenthood, up to 10% of pregnant women can become depressed at some point during pregnancy, says Dr. Channi Kumar at the Institute of Psychiatry in London.[95] Usually depression sets in during the first trimester (the first twelve weeks of pregnancy). Why?

First, the stress hormone cortisol doubles the first trimester, rising to about three times the normal level by the third trimester, say Deborah Sichel, MD, and Jeanne Watson Driscoll, co-authors of *Women's Moods*.[96] Some think these stress hormones could protect the baby from pregnancy stress and strengthen the mother–baby bond.

Second, estrogen and progesterone levels rise in the first trimester, and that increase can induce depressive symptoms. The levels of the hormone prolactin also increase to prepare the body for the formulation of mother's milk, and increased prolactin is associated with irritability and anger.

Anxiety, caused by hormonal shifts and possibly by the abnormal firing of synapses with norepinephrine, which triggers our fight-or-flight reflex, may also be a factor in first-trimester depression.

The brain may naturally accommodate these hormonal changes and work through morning sickness, so that expecting moms feel better in the second trimester (weeks twelve through twenty-six of the pregnancy).

Incidentally, fertility treatments can act in the limbic brain and produce severe depression, unstable moods, and sleep disruptions, as well as possibly reducing our ability to pay attention.

Brain Fog in Pregnancy

If you've been pregnant, you may remember that you couldn't remember anything.

Women in their third trimester experience forgetfulness approximately 15% more than the average person, found Wayne State University School of Medicine in Detroit.[97] Studies have yet to determine the reasons, but some hypotheses are:

High estrogen levels—more than 1,000 times *greater* than the levels at ovulation.

High level of oxytocin. The love hormone has an amnesic effect, which is great for childbirth, but makes it hard to be dazzlingly brilliant at work.

High levels of stress hormones—three times their normal amount. High levels of cortisol specifically may adversely affect the hippocampus, which plays a critical role in learning and memory.

Decreased brain-cell volume. Though your brain cell totals decrease in the third trimester, your brain will plump back up a few months after delivery.

Brain fog may encourage you to let go of the stressful world and get ready to nest. But the stressful world doesn't always want to let go. What helps?

- **Write down what you need to remember,** using white boards, sticky notes, and notebooks.

- **Create an information station,** one spot for all your time-organizing and communication materials.

- **Get appointment confirmations by email or text,** and mark down your appointments in your calendar or notebook.

- **Be a monotasker.** Do one thing, then the next thing.

- **Ask for help.** Your partner, older kids, and friends can help you remember what errands you need to do when.

- **Use your GPS** to get where you're going.

- **Rest yourself** and your brain.

- **Eat well** to keep your brain primed.

- **Exercise.**

- **Keep a sense of humor.**

Mom's Brain After Baby

Skipping right through childbirth (let's thank epidurals and the amnesiac hormone oxytocin, which gets released during labor), let's dive into a mother's postpartum brain.

The *baby blues* are not uncommon; 60 to 80% of new moms experience them after childbirth. The blues are unexpected sadness, crying, irritability, restlessness, and anxiety. They are similar to the pregnancy blues, but many women are jarred by having them while they have a new baby.

It makes sense that these blues occur when you consider all the changes new moms experience: a precipitous drop in estrogen and progesterone, fatigue from childbirth, the round-the-clock demands of the newborn, disappointment or guilt that things may not have gone as planned, the adjustment to breastfeeding, frustration about the still-poochy tummy, a messier house, and new negotiations with your partner.

Most times, baby blues fade in a couple of weeks as your body adjusts to the hormones and your new life. You may also learn how to function with less or interrupted rest. Meanwhile, it may help to:

> **Ask for and accept help,** even if it means adjusting your usual standards and habits a bit.
>
> **Focus on what's really important.** While a clean house may be relaxing, the effort to get it clean and keep it that way may just be too much for now. You, your baby, and your family are top of the list. Everything else is extra.
>
> **Eat well.** Keep cut veggies, fruit, cheese, sunflower or pumpkin seeds, and trail mix available. Eating these nutritious foods helps your blood sugar and mood.
>
> **Stay hydrated,** especially if you're nursing.
>
> **Take care of yourself.** Sleep when the baby's sleeping.
>
> **Be kind to yourself.** Being a parent means constant learning, mistakes, and growing—not perfection. If you constantly compare yourself to what you should do or

wish you could do, you miss out. Parenthood is a journey, not a destination, as they say.

Get dressed, so you like how you look.

Make sure your thyroid is still functioning well.

Treat yourself. A Netflix movie, ordering dinner with your partner while the baby sleeps, a long bath—do whatever helps you feel renewed.

Have a good laugh or good cry. It doesn't matter what you laugh or cry about. Both crying and laughing release tension from your body and change your perspective. Sad movies and comedies can trigger a good sob or deep belly laugh.

Go somewhere, at least once a day. Even a walk in the park, a visit to a mom's group, or a trip to the mall refreshes your view.

Move. From postpartum exercise or yoga to an exercise video, a walk, or dancing to old Madonna songs—all types of exercise help balance your hormones, boost your brain, and soothe your emotions.

When the baby blues don't abate within a month after childbirth and/or the symptoms seem to get worse, it's likely you have *postpartum depression (PPD),* which affects between 8 and 20% of women after pregnancy. Postpartum depression is a serious condition that can interfere with moms, the mom-baby relationship, and the family.

Postpartum depression can start soon after delivery or up to a year later, though it often occurs within the first four weeks after delivery. How long it lasts is different for every woman. Some women feel better in a few weeks; others may feel depressed for months or even a year or longer.

Symptoms are more pronounced than those of the baby blues and may include crying; irritability; insomnia; extreme fatigue; eating problems; persistent feelings of sadness, hopelessness, or helplessness; memory loss; and an inability or lack of desire to take care of yourself and/or your baby. Sometimes women suffering from PPD experience panic, mania, or even hallucinations or obsessive-compulsive thoughts or behaviors. In extreme cases, PPD can put the mom and baby's lives at risk.

Women who have a history of depression or anxiety have a higher chance of developing postpartum depression. So do those who abuse alcohol or other substances, smoke, experience a stressful pregnancy or stressful circumstance during pregnancy, are teens, had poor support or trauma in childhood, and/or get little support as a mother. These life experiences, say Sichel and Watson Driscoll in *Women's Moods, Women's Minds,* can set the stage for an emotional earthquake such as PPD or during other stressful hormonal events.[98]

If your baby blues don't improve, get worse, or simply interfere with daily life or cause concern, get support from your life partner and friends, and talk to a medical practitioner to sort out whether or not PPD may be making this time difficult.

Some of the same suggestions for the baby blues may help short-term with PPD. Eating fish for the omega-3 fatty acids may also help; however, one study found that taking fish-oil tablets during pregnancy didn't help with postpartum depression. Further research is needed to confirm the results.

Your practitioner may recommend a therapist to help treat your depression and/or antidepressants (there are some that are safe for breastfeeding mothers). Bright-light therapy has also been shown to reduce the symptoms of depression. You can also check with community centers, your medical office, neighborhood baby stores, and the Internet for support groups and places to turn for help.

The good thing is that PPD is one of the most treatable forms of depression. Remember you're not alone, and you can indeed get better.

The Adventure of Menopause

After you make it through pregnancy, your hormone levels go back to normal—at least for a little while. Then you have the adventure of menopause, when estrogen becomes the reclusive star everyone wants.

Menopause doesn't have an exact beginning, like your first period (menarche) or motherhood. Instead, menopause is defined in reverse, when you realize it's been a year since your last period. For most women, that's in the early fifties. *Perimenopause*—the transition from regular ovulation and menstruation to menopause—usually begins in the mid- to late-forties, but can start when you're thirty-five or so.

Lots of hormonal changes happen during perimenopause through post-menopause: the ovaries slowly stop making estrogen; meanwhile, the hypothalamus and pituitary gland stop reacting to the estrogen that's there.[99] Levels of estrogen and FSH decline dramatically, while other hormones, such as progesterone, testosterone, and other androgens decline more steadily.

Reactions to these changes—other than your menstrual cycle getting less predictable and then stopping—range from very few symptoms to the following: unexpected bursts of crankiness, broken nights of sleep, hair loss, vaginal dryness, skin changes, and even hearing loss. The most common concerns are mood swings and hot flashes, which happen as the brain goes through estrogen withdrawal.[100]

All these changes make the brain pretty tired.

Adjusting to a Different Brain

Laura, a psychologist and now almost sixty, noticed changes in her brain during perimenopause, which started in her late forties. She had trouble remembering, but worse was her brain fog: "It was as if I couldn't see my direction. Nothing seemed clear."

The biggest frustration was working with her therapy clients. As they talked, she'd think, "I know there is something intelligent I could say to bring all the pieces together, but I don't remember what that is." Instead, she shifted gears, becoming more of a nondirective therapist, listening and responding and then bringing her insights to the next session.

Laura took Remifemin, a standardized dose of the herb black cohosh used in Europe. It helped with her hot flashes and irritability, but not her cognition. But time helped. After a while, her memory came back, her hot flashes stopped, and her moods returned to normal.

If you've been in the same boat—perhaps asking yourself what you wanted when you came in the kitchen—here's what's happening: your brain depends solely on blood to function, and estrogen supports its blood supply. Less estrogen means less blood, so the brain gets smaller, especially in the hippocampus and parietal lobe, and the reduction possibly creates decreased mental clarity and short-term verbal-memory problems. On the other hand, interconnections between the neurons continue to grow.

> *Estrogen supports the brain's blood supply.*
> *Less estrogen means less blood to the brain,*
> *which may cause the mental-clarity and*
> *short-term verbal-memory problems*
> *that may be experienced in menopause.*

Christiane Northrup, MD, author of *Women's Bodies, Women's Wisdom,* believes that the brain changes that occur during menopause and aging may, in fact, make room for wisdom. "Brain cell loss with aging is akin to pruning the nonessential [neural] branches that may actually be interfering with optimal function," she says.[101]

We also miss estrogen because it affects the release of the neurotransmitter dopamine (affecting central nervous system, emotions, perceptions, and movement), serotonin (regulating mood, sleep, and learning), and norepinephrine (regulating stress, alertness, and arousal), according to the *Journal of Clinical Endocrinology & Metabolism.* The journal adds, "As estrogen levels decline over menopause, the cognitive and other behavioral processes that depend on them also decline, yet they appear to respond to estrogen replacement."[102]

If we replace the lost estrogen, can we reverse the aging process? And is replacing lost estrogen safe?

Hormone Replacement: Can Nature's Wonder Chemical Be Replaced?
The controversy about hormone replacement therapy (HRT) is worse than the one surrounding the 2000 George W. Bush–Al Gore presidential election results.

In HRT, also called hormone therapy or HT, women are given a combination of estrogen and progesterone, hormones that the body produces less of during menopause. These can be synthetic or derived from natural sources. Women who have had a hysterectomy and oophorectomy (removal of ovaries) also receive HRT, though we'll focus on age-related menopause here. Hormone replacement therapy has been prescribed as a treatment for:

- Hot flashes and night sweats;
- Vaginal dryness and pain with intercourse;
- Urinary tract infections;
- Interrupted sleep;
- Short-term memory difficulties;
- Osteoporosis and fractures;
- Lax pelvic floor muscles;
- Weakened muscle tone.

In 2000, Jane Brody from the *New York Times* said that HRT was "associated with a 50% reduction in heart disease and stroke." Preliminary research, she said, suggested that the risk of developing Alzheimer's disease was cut in half for those women who took estrogen for many years.[103] Over fifteen million women filled HRT prescriptions in one year—it was the thing to do.

But in 2002, the Women's Health Initiative (WHI) released a study of over 16,000 women who took estrogen plus progestin, a synthetic form of progesterone. Instead of getting the good results Brody cited, the study found that women were at *higher* risk for heart disease, blood clots, and breast cancer (but had *lower* risk of fractures and colon cancer). Adding fuel to the fire, in 2003, WHI reported that HRT may increase the risk of stroke and dementia.[104] That put the brakes on HRT prescriptions.

But science is ever-changing. In the past decade, the WHI study was studied (as it were) for factors besides HRT that may have influenced the results. For instance, many of the participants were in their sixties, with thirteen years between when they experienced menopause and when they received HRT. Would results have been different if the women had started HRT earlier? Did the type of HRT make a difference? Or would other combinations of estrogen with progestin (synthetic progesterone) or estrogen alone work better?

Other questions about hormone therapy and menopause take an even broader tact: Did the women in the WHI study have a vitamin D deficiency, which can increase the risk of breast cancer? Can excess fat change the production of hormones and the body's response to them? What's the interaction between hormones and higher-risk behaviors, like smoking or excess drinking?[105]

Bio-identical Hormones: Can We Duplicate Nature?

Bio-identical hormones are based on compounds found in plants. They are processed into an individualized dosage by a compounding pharmacist. Just like synthetic hormones, bio-identical ones are formulated to stabilize hormone levels and lessen menopausal symptoms.

Many say these bio-identical hormones are more compatible with and molecularly identical to human hormones—compared to the HRT hormones created by pharmaceutical companies. Others say that's absolutely not true.

It is unknown if bio-identical hormones are safer than synthetic ones, because there have been no large studies done on bio-identical hormones. The theory is that there's little incentive to conduct such studies, since they're usually funded by the pharmaceutical companies, which can't patent bio-identical hormones and, therefore, don't want to pay for such research.

Many people see bio-identical hormones as a valuable, underappreciated resource suppressed by big pharmaceuticals. Many others see them as unregulated, risky products with unsubstantiated claims. If you consider using bio-identical hormones for help with hormonal changes, spend some

The U.S. Food and Drug Administration (FDA) is now suggesting women can use HRT to treat menopausal symptoms for a short period of time, with the lowest dose possible. And recent research shows that low-dosage patches significantly reduce women's risk of stroke.[106]

The latest medical recommendations, given in the *British Medical Journal* and elsewhere, encourage women to begin HRT within the first five to six years after menopause, though questions about HRT's effects on potential breast cancer linger.

time to research on your own, taking the extreme points of view with a grain of salt.

Naturopathic doctor Eileen Stretch prescribes bio-identical hormone treatment to patients who are not served by changes in diet or other treatments. She gives the smallest effective dose to each individual patient for the symptoms. "I'm not trying to get women back to where they were twenty years ago," she says.

She almost always recommends vaginal estrogen, a suppository that's absorbed in the vaginal tract. It helps prevent changes in the vagina, including dryness that can result in less accurate pap smears, more frequent urinary tract infections, and inner labia atrophy—changes in the size of the inner or minor labia, the folds or lips closest to the vaginal opening. It also can help with sex. An eighty-nine-year-old patient had painful sex when she became involved with a younger boyfriend in his seventies. Stretch prescribed vaginal estrogen. The patient reported that sex was delightful, with some of the best orgasms of her life. (And sex is good for the brain.)

Sherree couldn't predict what might happen to her body and brain over the next fifteen to twenty years, but she decided she could do things to prepare for menopause.

First, she focused on the good-for-you things that would help her now as well as set the stage for the future—exercise, for one. She developed a habit of moving hard at least three times a week. And the next time she went for a pap smear, she talked to her doctor about hormones, thinking she'd feel less freaked out about her choices if she learned about them in advance. She also asked for a test to see if she was in perimenopause and discussed supplements.

In the end, she still wasn't looking forward to the change, but she had learned she could handle menopause, and might even get a little wiser in the process.

Chapter 5

The Dance of Your Body and Brain

Sometimes your body is smarter than you are.

Anonymous

The sea squirt plant starts as a larva with a rudimentary brain (about 300 neurons compared to humans' 50 to 100 billion). It travels to the shallow waters until it finds a place to put down roots. Then, with no more need for the brain, the larva eats it.[107] Yum!

Moving things need brains, but brains also need movement. "Movement is fundamental to the very existence of the brain. All our higher levels of thinking, our cognitive abilities, emerged from the motor system," says John Ratey, MD, author of *Spark: The Revolutionary New Science of Exercise and the Brain.*[108]

In addition to supporting our brains, movement helps our bodies get slimmer, grow stronger, sleep better, maintain strong bones, breathe better, build the heart, and combat chronic diseases, such as diabetes, high blood pressure, arthritis, and certain types of cancer. Not a bad list. But, "building muscles and conditioning the heart and lungs are essentially side effects," says Ratey. "I often tell my patients that the point of exercise is to build and condition the brain."[109]

Exercise benefits the brain well beyond the runner's high (the release of neurotransmitter endorphins). During exercise, your body also releases other hormones and increases the levels of oxygenated blood that reach the brain—all of which helps with mood, depression, and anxiety.[110] But exercise also creates and protects new neurons, strengthens connections between them, and increases the number of branches (dendrites) used to make those connections. In other words, movement helps make your brain smarter.

*Moving your body actually helps make you smarter,
because movement positively affects
the brain's neurons and neural pathways.*

A side note here about the word *exercise:* it's full of *shoulds, have tos,* and *not enoughs.* It brings to mind the sneers of my former gym teacher, Miss Joann, "Is that *all* you can do?" Think about this: People don't as happily say, "I'm going to exercise." Instead they have more excitement as they describe themselves *moving:* "I'm going to run/walk/bike/skate/play Frisbee/swim/use the treadmill/work out at the gym."

Move is a whole different word. It's what the body is doing as it stretches, walks, jumps, pulls, pushes, goes through space, and uses its muscles. What a gift! You don't have to be aerobic to feel benefits: even just a little movement throughout the day enhances weight loss and maintains health.[111] But when you move enough to feel your body heat up, you add a level of aliveness in your body and brain—even your cells move with the flow.

I'll use the word *exercise* because it's convenient, but what I really mean is *moving*—especially *moving intensely, moving hard.*

Our bodies and brains are partners in movement and change. The more you support that partnership, the happier both will be. Any movement you do—from exercise to smiling and singing—helps your brain.

Exercising Your Brain
(Without Opening a Book)

The Naperville, Illinois school system instituted a brand new physical education program in the late 1990s. Instead of subjecting kids to dodge ball games or climbing ropes, the program incorporated activities such as kayaking, square dancing, and rock climbing—just about anything that raised the heart rate into the target zone for cardiovascular fitness. The aim? To teach kids how to be fit throughout life.

The new program produced good health results: only 3% of students in this school system are overweight, compared to 30% nationally. But the happy surprise was that the physical education program increased the school's academic scores. The Naperville school system rose to the top tier of Illinois schools in academic testing, despite spending considerably less per student than the other school systems it bested. On top of that, it scored highest in the world in science on the recognized Trends in International Mathematics and Science Study test; they scored sixth in the world in math.[112]

Other schools and research have confirmed what Naperville experienced. For instance, the California Department of Education found that students with higher fitness scores have higher test scores.

Better physical fitness means better attention and better learning.

Exercise can physically bolster your brain's infrastructure.

Exercise, Ratey points out, can also reverse both the brain shrinkage caused by depression and the disconnection of brain cells caused by toxic stress. "Exercise unleashes a cascade of neurochemicals and growth factors that can physically bolster the brain's infrastructure," he says. "In fact, the brain responds like muscles do, growing with use, withering with inactivity."[113]

Exercise tells your brain to release a family of proteins called *factors* that build and maintain cell circuitry. The most important one is brain-derived neurotrophic factor (BDNF), which supports the survival and growth of neurons. BDNF helps neurons automatically sprout new branches in the synapses—the structural growth needed for learning. This Miracle-Gro for the brain also:

- Improves signal strength between neurons;
- Directs "traffic" along neuropathways and engineers the pathways themselves;
- Improves the functions of neurons, encourages their growth, and strengthens and protects them against the natural process of cell death;

- Activates genes that help produce *more* BDNF, serotonin, and other proteins that build synapses.[114]

You get BDNF from learning and exercise.

Exercise floods the brain, particularly the *hippocampus* (which regulates emotion, navigation, and memory) with BDNF. That's why exercise makes you feel better and increases your rate of learning. In one study, people learned vocabulary words 20% faster following exercise than they did before working out. Exercise can change the chemical composition of your hippocampus, according to a recent University of New South Wales study. It optimizes alertness, attention, and motivation; helps nerve cells bind together; and spurs the stem cells in the hippocampus to develop new nerve cells.[115]

Exercise alone won't make you *smarter*, points out Carl Cotman, the researcher who pioneered research on the link between BDNF and exercise.[116] Learning itself means you respond to something in a different way. But BDNF gives you something *more* to respond with. As the Naperville physical education coordinator put it, "In our department, we create brain cells. It's up to the other teachers to fill them."

Exercise Helps You Deal

Exercise does more than improve learning. When you really move, you give yourself benefits affecting your mood, addiction, aging, and more. When you exercise, you:

Grow your brain. As mentioned earlier, exercise massively increases neurogenesis—new neuron growth.[117]

Reduce stress. Exercise calms the body and counters the influence of cortisol, the stress hormone.

Create calm and confidence. Rigorous exercise interrupts the anxiety feedback loop to the brain;[118] reduces muscle tension; modulates serotonin, norepinephrine, and GABA (a calming neurotransmitter); helps you change your perception of fear into something more handleable, like excitement; allows you to move rather than hide; and improves resilience.[119]

Reduce depression. Physical activity increases endorphins (elevating mood); counteracts cortisol (reducing stress); regulates the same neurotransmitters targeted by antidepressants, such as norepinephrine (which activates the brain), dopamine (which jump-starts attention and motivation), and serotonin (which improves mood, impulse control, and self-esteem).[120]

Add focus. Exercise helps with attention-deficit disorder (ADD) and attention-deficit hyperactivity disorder (ADHD) because it increases dopamine and norepinephrine, which help the centers for refocus (basal ganglia)[121] and attention (locus coeruleus).

Make choices versus acting from compulsion. Just ten minutes of exercise has been shown to blunt an alcohol craving, and five minutes of intense exercise can fend off the craving for a cigarette.[122] Exercise produces *endocannabinoids,* a neurotransmitter that mimics the effects of morphine and THC, with no withdrawal effects.

Smooth monthly cycles. Moving intensely increases the amount of tryptophan that pushes through the blood-brain barrier, which in turn increases concentrations of serotonin in the brain.

Ease pregnancy. Exercise lowers stress, improves mood, can reduce nausea, and can possibly improve the brain development of the baby. It also helps counter the effects of hormonal changes that lead to postpartum depression.

Improve menopause. Exercise protects against heart disease, diabetes, breast cancer, cognitive decline, and stroke. "Exercise tricks the brain into trying to maintain itself for survival, despite the hormonal cues that it is aging," says Ratey in his book *Spark.*[123]

Slow aging. Moving hard increases our adaptability to stress, blood flow to brain, neurogenesis (cell production), brain volume in hippocampus and the frontal and temporal lobes, and neurotrophic factors that possibly slow the effect of Alzheimer's. It also reduces inflammation and fosters neuroplasticity.[124]

It's Not What You Know; It's What You Do

None of this information about the benefits of exercise actually laces up your shoes and gets you running. Only half of Americans exercise for thirty minutes three times a week,[125] so odds are you could use more exercise.

Dr. Rosemary Agostini, medical chief of the Activity, Sports, and Exercise Medicine Department at Group Health Cooperative in Seattle, is an expert at getting patients of all ages and all stages to move. Her first step starts with moving more; in fact, the Mayo Clinic is studying positive effects of extra movements, called "non-exercise activity thermogenesis" (NEAT), such as:

- Swearing off the elevator for a week, or even getting off one floor below your destination.
- Walking with friends instead of sitting for coffee with them.
- Holding work meetings as you and your coworkers walk around the block.
- Pacing when you're cogitating on an idea.

The next step is to do a little more, again. Increase your movement for the next week. Then, when you're ready to intentionally exercise, Agostini suggests focusing on four things: fun, purpose, community, and kindness.

Fun: Come up with activities and ways to exercise that are enjoyable. If you don't like to be sweaty, try deep water aerobics. If you like music, try a dance class.

Purpose: Create meaning from what you do. Become engaged in an athletic event that helps raise money for a cause. Try walking or running a five- or ten-kilometer race or a hiking or biking event. Many such events provide support, coaches, and a community to give you momentum. You can also write down your motivation, such as "I want to be able to play with my grandchildren," on your fridge or make it the phrase that you see when you make a call on your cell phone. Or you can find meaning by rewarding yourself. For example, every time you exercise, put a dollar or five dollars in a jar to save for something special, like a trip to Hawaii.

Community: You don't have to do this exercise thing all by yourself. Get a workout buddy. Find a trainer who motivates you to follow through for the week. If you exercise at work, "chances are higher you'll keep with it," says Agostini.

Kindness: Be gentle with your lovely self. Stop the bullying ("I should exercise"), and start being compassionate to yourself. Make your increments of success small and accomplishable. "If I only have ten minutes, I do ten minutes, and that's fabulous," says Agostini.

But Agostini does suggest that, to be fit, you get active at least thirty minutes a day, four days a week. The American Heart Association's website explains how to determine and monitor your target heart rate. Once you've done that, find ways to gently push yourself—even just increasing your pace for a few minutes several times during your exercise session.

Stress Is Actually Accenting the Wrong Syllable

Want to get all wound up? Let's talk about too much stress: the ambulance screaming behind you when the road is jammed, the microwave that breaks as you're getting dinner ready, the teen who brought home a report card with two F's, the important call you can't pick up because you don't know which button to press on your new cell phone.

It's not that you don't want *any* stress. With just enough stress, your brain releases norepinephrine, which at healthy levels, makes you happy, helps create new memories, and is a general exciter agent for your brain. Stressful situations will feel more like rewarding challenges if you're at the right stress level.

But with too much stress, your body and brain suffer. Physically, you may experience sleep disturbances, muscle tension, headache, digestive problems, and fatigue. Emotionally, you might have nervousness, anxiety, a loss of enthusiasm or energy, and mood changes. Stress-related behaviors include changed eating habits (over- or undereating, binge eating, or other poor eating habits), irritability, anger, and a need for control. They might also include addictive activities, such as alcohol or drug abuse and smoking.

From the point of view of the brain and nervous system, stress equals high alert. The brain tells your adrenal glands to release the hormone adrenaline; the hypothalamus relays signals through the pituitary gland, then the adrenal cortex, to produce cortisol, the stress hormone. These hormonal changes trigger the fight-or-flight response of the sympathetic nervous system.[126] Adrenaline and cortisol keep your primary responses geared up; they raise blood sugar and blood pressure, dilate pupils, and increase breathing and heart rates. And they shut down peripheral responses, including sexual and immune-system functions. They even trigger the release of the bladder and anal sphincter. They also make the blood-brain barrier less effective, so neurons are more exposed to some toxins and viruses.

Like a leaky faucet, the sympathetic nervous system is hard to turn off. It keeps itself turned on for self-protection. After a near-miss car accident in traffic, you become overly attentive to cars for the rest of the drive home. But if high alerts become chronic stress, you kill brain cells with overexcitement and become susceptible to a variety of symptoms, such as gum disease, backaches, anxiety and mood swings, rashes, poor concentration, stomach problems, varicose veins, and even suicidal thoughts.

On the other side, your body balances stress with the parasympathetic nervous system. It has hormones that want to rest and digest. They do so by curbing the release of cortisol and gathering its leftovers from the brain, lowering your heart rate and blood pressure, and re-engaging the digestive system.

But you don't have to wait for the parasympathetic nervous system to kick in to stop stressing out. Much of our stress comes from our worries and expectations, rather than from real physical dangers. Right now, in this very moment, you can find calm, warmth, safety, and satisfaction.

Internal Antistress Responses

While we often blame stress on what happens to us, we can reduce our stress on our own. The first way is moving hard, because exercise gets you tapped back into life—not your mind.

- Exercise stresses your brain in a good way, activating and strengthening the same neural pathways you use to deal with life stress, like looking for a job or remodeling your bathroom.
- It helps your cells recover after being immersed in cortisol, which can turn into belly fat when it hangs around. (However, the fears about belly fat and certain heart problems have been reexamined lately.)
- It also releases cortisol—again because you're stressing your body. But as you continue to train and exercise, your body becomes better able to deal with both physical and emotional stress and decrease the need to release cortisol.[127] In other words, exercise calms the body so it can handle stress more easily.
- It releases BDNF, which can help you learn a new way to deal with your stressors.

Beyond movement or exercise, here are other ways you can change your responses to stress:

- Come back to your body and senses in this very moment. It is often a gentler experience than hanging out in your stressed mind.
- Drink water.
- Eat fish or take fish oil. (For more food suggestions, see chapter 8.)
- Say no. Choose and follow your priorities, even in the give-and-take of life. Do what's needed, not what you feel you should do.
- Be kind to yourself.
- Consider whether or not what's stressing you now will really matter in five years. If not, treat it less intensely.
- Remind your worried and anxious self that you are a good person, doing a good job taking care of what's really important and of yourself.
- Be grateful.
- Remember that the bigger part of life continues no matter what.

External Changes to Stress

Change what's bugging you—even for a little while.

- Reduce stimulation from electronics, unending news, and clutter.
- Reduce stimulation from your family! Take a break.
- Find or create a quiet(er) spot.
- Meditate. Feel the forces that make you breathe and keep you alive; you don't have to do anything.
- Be creative.
- Get in touch with the natural world.
- And move. Pace, stretch, lift an exercise ball, even wiggle your foot.

Go to Bed: Sleep

"Sleep deprivation is the most common brain impairment," says William Dement, noted author of *The Promise of Sleep*.[128] Brains need downtime, but with work deadlines, screaming babies, lights and Internet connections 24/7, the world does not easily let go. Add to that caffeine, stress, and fear of insomnia ("I *have to* sleep, damn it!"), and it's easy to consider sleep and rest as an extra treat, not a necessity.

When you don't get enough sleep, your brain has to work harder to compensate.[129] Emotionally, a sleep-deprived brain dramatically overreacts to negative experiences. On the one hand, short-term sleep deprivation doesn't significantly impact your executive functioning abilities—your working memory and ability to process information. But it *does* significantly distort your information intake, according to a study where subjects didn't sleep for fifty-one hours.[130]

Here are more things that happen to you when your brain wants to rest; they can be triggered by a short-term lack of sleep or ongoing sleep deprivation:

- A reduced ability to focus and complete tasks;
- Problems with concentration and memory;

- Irritability, edginess, discomfort, and a lower threshold for stress;
- Anxiety disorders;
- Slower reaction times;
- Blurred vision;
- Depression;
- Alterations in appetite;
- Heart disease;
- Hallucinations;
- Frequent infections;
- Behavioral, learning, or social problems.

Sleep can help regulate the hormones governing hunger.[131] When you suffer sleep deprivation, levels of leptin (a hormone that makes us feel full and satisfied) fall while levels of ghrelin (which stimulates appetite) increase.[132] So you keep eating and never feel satisfied.

Here are some ways to get deep rest—perhaps leading to sleep. They are taken from my book *Restful Insomnia: How to Get the Benefits of Sleep, Even When You Can't:*

- Start by creating a dusk—withdrawing from the world, turning off lights, getting the house and yourself ready for bed—about an hour or two before bedtime.
- Lower the lights (darkness stimulates the production of melatonin).
- Reduce electronic interactions.
- Create a dark and comfortable place to rest and sleep.
- Bring your focus back to your body sensations, to give less energy to your thoughts.

If you suspect you have a sleeping problem, check with your doctor. You may have sleep apnea or another illness that requires treatment, or you may find help by using cognitive behavioral therapy to get back in sleep rhythm.

Enjoy Sex

Your brain savors sex as much as your body does. The physical activity of sex delivers more blood and oxygen to the brain. The multisensory experience stimulates the brain.[133] Sex increases neurogenesis (the growth of neurons) and connections between brain cells, as discovered by Princeton researchers.[134] They also found that sex reduces anxiety. In fact, during sexual activity, the parts of the female brain associated with processing fear, anxiety, and emotion relax, and during orgasm, they almost close down.[135] During orgasm, the brain releases neurohormones oxytocin and vasopressin, which both act as analgesics (pain relievers).[136]

If half-naked buff men jogging in the park do not spark your sexual urges, the Internet has nurtured sexual sites (beyond the 1.5 billion sites rated XXX) that support a woman's point of view. Here are a few:

- Women-owned Babeland *(www.babeland.com),* which sells sex toys and DVDs for men and women;

- Oysters and Chocolate *(www.oystersandchocolate. com),* erotica stories and images;

- *About.com*'s discussion of sex and older women.[137]

As Carl Jung said, "The brain is viewed as an appendage of the genital glands." If you have orgasm or don't, increasing your sexual experience helps the brain. Feel your sexy self.

Go Ahead, *Y-a-w-n*

Even though yawning is considered rude, especially if you make others yawn, go ahead, yawn away. It makes brains happier. We think of yawning as a sign of boredom or sleepiness, but fetuses yawn at twenty weeks after conception, and it's unlikely that they're bored already! Some birds and reptiles as well as most mammals yawn, though yawning is infectious only among great apes, macaque monkeys, chimpanzees, and humans. Even just reading about yawning makes you want to. Have you yawned yet?

While the reasons for yawning are still a mystery in many ways, we do know that yawning:

- Stimulates the brain and makes you more alert, rather than making you more sleepy.

- Regulates the temperature and metabolism of the brain.

- Optimizes brain activity.

- Stimulates alertness and concentration.

- Improves cognitive function and memory recall.

- Relaxes the body.

- Reduces stress.

- Fine-tunes circadian rhythms.

- Increases empathy.

- Enhances pleasure and sensuality.

"It's hard to find another activity that positively influences so many functions of the brain," says Andrew Newberg, MD, author of *How God Changes Your Brain.*[138]

Yawning positively influences many brain functions.

To invigorate your brain, yawn as often as you can during the day—as you wake, before you sleep, when you're confronting a problem, when you're feeling stress. And go for a full yawn work-out, which makes you feel "utterly present, incredibly relaxed, and highly alert," says Newberg. All you have to do is fake it. Pretend to yawn six or seven times, and a real one will begin to emerge. Keep going for another six or seven, until you move through a wave of yawning. In less than a minute, you'll provide your brain with a neurological delight.

Laughter and Smiling

Laughter and smiling—regardless of whether they are triggered by a Tina Fey character or Jon Stewart skewering Congress—positively affects the body and the brain. For instance, laughter:

- Reduces the level of stress hormones such as cortisol, epinephrine, and adrenaline,
- Increases the levels endorphins, feel-good hormones,
- Increases neurotransmitter connections in your brain,
- Helps your immune system stay strong by both increasing the number of antibody-producing cells and enhancing the efficiency of your T-cells.

A good belly laugh also exercises the diaphragm, contracts the abs, and works out the shoulders. A hundred laughs are equivalent to fifteen minutes on the exercise bike, or so it's said. Laughter yoga and laughter groups use the infectious nature of laughter to create a cacophony of glee.

What is happening in your brain when you just have to chuckle? Your neural network, in both the frontal and temporal regions, regulates the perception of humor. We all have developed different networks and find different things funny. When something strikes you as hilarious, your brain networks induce facial reactions. It starts with smiles, and if the humor is really funny, the brainstem gets the laughter going.

Smiling ain't so bad for the brain, either. Smiling helps your mood and attitude become more positive, and it reduces stress. Smiling helps you release more endorphins and enkephalins (the body's natural painkillers),[139] as well as serotonin (which regulates mood, appetite, sleep, and some cognitive functions).

Smiling also encourages more kind and generous responses to others. It is a contagious expression, like yawning and laughing, and helps you connect better, which in turn, stimulates the brain. A smile helps you look younger and feel healthier as it lowers your blood pressure and boosts the activities of your immune system.[140]

> *Smiling helps you connect with others,*
> *look younger, and feel healthier.*

Researchers at several universities, including Temple University in Philadelphia, have explored how different kinds of smiles create different emotional responses.[141] They compared a full facial smile versus the smile using just the mouth (you know, the Miss America smile that creates no eye wrinkles).[142] Those with a full smile reported more positive emotions and had increased attentional flexibility: they could attend to and switch focus between attributes more easily.

Even a teensy smile makes a difference. Vietnamese Buddhist monk Thich Nhat Han suggests creating a half smile—think of Mona Lisa's expression—when you wake, meditate, are irritated, listen to music, or just have a free moment. The Inner Smile meditation comes from Healing Tao: think of something or someone who will make you smile, then imagine sending that smile all through your body from the center of your brain down through your throat and digestive system to your toes.

Smiling and laughter won't keep your sweetie from cheating or stop company layoffs. But they will help your brain function better and widen your perspectives.

Sense Your World

Humans experience the world through the five senses: sight, smell, touch, sound, and taste. Every moment, those five senses work together to deliver the play-by-play of your reality. They team up to tell your brain what's going on. For example:

Sight: Dog on the bed,

Smell: Funky,

Touch: Nappy,

Sound: Panting,

Taste: Well, you don't need all the senses to get the message.

Working together, the senses alert your brain that it's time to shoo that dog off your bed and make an appointment at the groomer's.

One way to stimulate your brain is through your sensory systems, which are considered by many to be the "windows to the brain." Lawrence C. Katz, PhD, a professor of neurobiology at Duke University Medical Center, developed a series of brain exercises that uses the senses in unexpected ways.[143] Using your senses, he says, helps your brain manufacture nutrients that strengthen, preserve, and grow brain cells.

To include one or more of your senses in an everyday task, try:

- Getting dressed with your eyes closed.
- Rubbing your cheek with a flower petal.
- Noticing silence between the sounds you hear.
- Wearing earplugs while playing music, so you feel the vibrations instead of hearing the sounds.
- Sharing a meal with another person and using only visual cues—no talking—to communicate your experience.

To combine senses, try:

- Listening to music and smelling flowers.
- Listening to falling rain and tapping your fingers,
- Watching clouds while playing with modeling clay.

Your senses are your brain's avenue to experience, learn from, and remember the world. So go out and take a look, give a listen, get a whiff, taste some samples, and reach out and touch the playground you live in—even if you encounter a few smelly doggies on the way.

Cushion the Brain

A knock on the head used to be ignored in high school football. "Tough it out and play!" coaches would say. No one—except the child's mom, most likely—noticed changes that could happen after a head injury: confusion, headaches, blurred vision, memory loss, neck pain, weakness or numbness in limbs, nausea, coordination, and emotional reactions, such as anxiety and irritability. Serious traumatic brain injury (TBI) or multiple concussions can lead to chronic brain damage, which in turn can lead to depression, memory loss, speech impediments, erratic behavior, hallucinations, and even dementia.[144] When the brain gets hurt, it doesn't get bruised as much as violently shaken, which is why whiplash creates problems. The brain cells become depolarized and fire their neurotransmitters, said the *New York Times* in an October 10, 2010, online article, "Head Injuries in Football." The brain, flooded with chemicals, can burn out certain learning and memory receptors.[145]

Fortunately, many states have legislated rules so children and adolescent athletes get care to recover from a concussion. Even if you don't spend much time on a football field, you can be vulnerable to brain injury from sports, falls, violence, and accidents. The Brain Injury Association says that each year, 140,000 persons die from brain injuries, and 70,000 persons sustain severe brain injuries. The website *Sixwise.com,* which collects health and safety advice from experts, offers the following tips for protecting your brain.[146]

Be Safe in Cars and Around Cars

- Chose the safest car—meaning the car most likely to prevent injuries—and one with airbags. Use lap and shoulder belts.

- Don't use a cell phone while driving—either for calls or texting. You're four times more likely to have an accident when you do, according to the road safety campaign in Britain. Even using a headset, you're distracted as much as if you were over the legal blood-alcohol limit.

- Wear bright, reflective clothing when walking, especially after dark. Use crosswalks, but keep alert when you do.

- Don't use cell phones when walking, either. Studies at Rutgers show that pedestrian deaths are higher for people talking on the phone while they're on foot.

Wear Bicycle and Motorcycle Helmets

- Wear a dorky helmet. In 2009, 51,000 bicyclists were injured in traffic.[147] Nearly 80% of fatal bicycle crashes are due to head injuries. Helmets are 85 to 88% effective in preventing head injuries, according to the National Highway Traffic Safety Administration. Helmets should fit directly over your forehead and have tight chinstraps.

- Without a helmet, motorcyclists are fourteen times more likely to die in a crash and three times more likely to incur a head injury.

- If your helmet hits a hard surface—in an accident or if you drop it down the stairs—it loses its ability to absorb the shock of a hard blow. Time for a new one.

Stay Upright, Keep Steady

Falls are the leading cause of head injuries for the elderly, but even agile younger folks need to stay safe.

- Exercise to maintain strength and balance.

- Keep floors uncluttered. Especially keep electrical cords out of the way and avoid loose rugs. Install grab-bars in your bathroom.

- Stay upright in rain and snow: skid-proof your stairs, carry fewer items during wet weather, wear sturdy boots, and even use walking sticks to keep your balance.

Protect Yourself

Violence is an often-unmentioned threat to women's brains. Protect yourself from violence by taking self-defense courses and identifying warning signs and precursors to violence. "Real fear is a gift because it is a survival signal that sounds in the presence of danger," says Gavin de Becker, author of *The Gift of Fear*. "If you turn it off, you won't be informed when you are in danger. Unwarranted fear is a waste of time; it's destructive."

e͜ɔ

Movement is life. Because you have a brain, you can move. Relish anything you can do to move, and see if you can find ways to move more. Moving is a gift that helps you verify the joy and experience of being alive.

Chapter 6

Creative Learning _____
All Work and No Play Gives Jane a Dull Brain

I am not young enough to know everything.

Oscar Wilde, playwright

It was a small car collision. Nothing was broken, the car was repaired, but the accident shook Renna's world—shook her brain, actually.

Renna began to forget. She forgot where she was driving until she checked what she had put in the car. She typed the wrong words in the stories she wrote. She couldn't read adult books, just ones written for kids. Her business was a mess—she didn't know if she'd delivered the products she was sending invoices for. "My short-term memory was useless," she told me years later.

The doctors thought her problem was age (she was fifty), but Renna was sure her memory loss stemmed from the car accident. The docs finally administered tests and a CAT scan and then admitted Renna had cognitive difficulty. Whiplash could be the cause.

Having the problem confirmed didn't make her problems disappear. "I had to figure out how to fix myself," she said.

Years before, Renna had written an article about chickadees growing new brain cells. "If birds can do it," she decided, "so can I." The first step was brain exercise to regenerate her memory. The key was learning something new.

To her surprise, math tweaked her imagination, despite her math anxiety. Renna had taken the easiest math class in high school, hated balancing her checkbook, and let friends figure out tips. She wasn't interested in calculating the square root of 1,912,689, but Renna connected to math through fairy tales, tarot, and astrology. She'd add in her head how many fairies were in the original Sleeping Beauty story. She noticed the number patterns in tarot. She created astrology charts without using calculators, much less computers.

As her brain regained its abilities, she played with math in daily life, averaging the number of people in lines at the grocery store and multiplying numbers on license plates. She eventually wrote a book about what she learned, *Math for Mystics.* Math reignited her brain.

Even if you don't need to restore your memory, you still want to be sharp, if only to stay on top of our daily deluge of information. Staying sharp gets harder as you get older, and not because we lose brain cells. The older you are, the less time you have to keep up with new technology. And you have more information to remember—from last year's sales figures to what your niece likes for her birthday.

You also have more wisdom taking up room in your brain. The University of California in San Diego says wisdom is the ability to make the best use of knowledge. Brainwise, wisdom is your advanced cognitive and emotional development, driven by your experience.[148]

You can support yourself in order to stay on top of learning, information, and names. As you keep your brain plastic, flexible, and agile, you are getting a boost to excel in the busy world.

The Plastic, Elastic Brain

Veronica ate breakfast while her son, Cameron, worked on last-minute homework. "Mom," he said. "You aced math in high school. Can you help me with this?"

"Um . . . sure," she replied as she leaned over to look at the problem. Sine, cosine, and tangent functions—she remembered doing them, but she didn't remember how, even after looking at the chapter instructions in Cameron's math book. What had happened to her math smarts?

The smarts didn't disappear—they morphed. Math in high school helped her brain become a better learning machine. But since she didn't maintain her math connections, her brain reused and recycled those neurons to help her learn law, French, and even how to be a better parent.

Your plastic brain can rearrange itself, something first discovered in 1820. Nearly two centuries later, scientists at the Massachusetts Institute of Technology found that neurons didn't just rearrange, but they were also multifunctional. The researchers took the optic nerves in the brain of a ferret and rewired them to the auditory cortex—and then those auditory nerves were used for seeing.[149]

Neurons not only rearrange themselves, but they're also multifunctional.

If you could stick a little camera in your brain, you'd see immense physical changes going on as neural connections were made and remade. The brain's gray (thinking) matter thickens or shrinks as neural connections build and weaken. When you create a memory to learn someone's name at a party, you form new neural connections. Later, when you've forgotten that name, those same connections are weakened or reused for a different purpose.

Practice will keep those neural connections "oiled." If Veronica had periodically done a few cofunctions or graphing ratios, or if she'd brushed up with a few days' practice, she could have helped Cameron with math.

Plastic brains are also what cause phantom limb pain—when someone who lost an arm or leg still feels the limb hurt or itch. The phantom pain may happen because the neurons that used to track pain in the arm have been reused for another body part—the face, eye, or ear. When the ear hurts, the person thinks it's her arm that's hurting because she doesn't know the brain has recycled neurons from the arm.

The good news is your brain keeps growing. In fact, it does not stop changing from the day you're born until the day you die.

Our brains always keep growing. From the day we're born until the day we die, they are always changing.

New skills change our brain maps, neural pathways, and hundreds of millions and possibly billions of the connections between the nerve cells, says Michael Merzenich, a University of California San Francisco neuroscientist who's changed the way the scientific community looks at the brain.[150] Not only can we train our brains to learn different skills, he says, but the more we do it, the faster our brains will process information and the more efficient our neurons will become—at learning, solving cognitive problems, processing emotions, and even treating brain disorders.

Forget to Remember

No matter how much you practice remembering, the brain is still built to forget. If you remembered everything (every phone number you've ever heard, every background conversation at the coffee shop, every word problem in middle school algebra), your brain would overload, and you'd have a hard time setting priorities about what's really important. (A rare few people have extraordinary autobiographical memory, which creates its own challenges.) Your brain prunes knowledge so it's easier to get to the most useful information you need now.

Stanford University researchers wanted to figure out how forgetting happens. They found that the prefrontal cortex tells the hippocampus (responsible for creating, storing, and retrieving memory) to *not* remember a specific task.[151]

So let's have some sympathy for your memory. It works hard but rarely gets a break, which is a chance to make connections stick. Your brain gets more chances with meditation, rest, sleep, and even play.

You Must Remember This

If forgetting is part of nature, what about remembering? Remembering is not just a passive habit.

The first place you store memories is in your *short-term* or *working memory*. Seven is its lucky number—the maximum pieces of information it can hold for ten to twenty seconds. If the short-term information is something you can practice or if you can link it to what you already know, you can transfer it into your *long-term memory.* Long-term memory is the ability to recall sensations, events, ideas, and other information for long periods of time without apparent effort.

Memory functions as a continuum. From easiest to hardest to forget, you have:

> **Semantic** memories, your concepts and factual knowledge;
>
> **Procedural** memory to learn new skills and acquire habits;
>
> **Episodic** memory, when you recall personal incidents;
>
> **Automatic** memory, or memory made from habit;
>
> **Reflexive/conditioned** memory, or memories created by the hot stove effect;
>
> **Reflexive/emotional** memory, when emotions and beliefs trigger memories, such as details about your son leaving for overnight camp as he packs for college.

To help trigger your memory, start with your body. When information is all theoretical, it goes in and out of the head. Your senses are gateways to storing and accessing information. Seeing, hearing, smelling, and tasting help you use the whole brain, giving you more memory roots to tap into. Create an image or a soundtrack to something you want to remember. When you've forgotten what you're looking for in the basement, follow your nose—you body knows where it wants to go, even if you've temporarily forgotten why.

Emotions are also key to the memory process. Do you have a detailed memory from September 11, 2001, when Barack Obama was elected president, or when Michael Jackson died? Early childhood memories are often tied to strong emotions—the stronger the emotion, the stronger the imprint on your senses.

As mentioned earlier, practice lubricates your new neural pathways, making it easier and easier to do what you're learning. Movement also helps etch memories. The cerebellum (involved with voluntary motor movement, balance and equilibrium, and muscle tone) combines movement messages with visual and auditory ones and relays them back and forth to the cortex. That message transfer stimulates growth in both the moving and thinking brains.[152]

Exercising, especially if you do it before you learn, helps release a learning "fertilizer," brain-derived neurotrophic factors (BDNF), as mentioned in chapter 5, to help your connections grow.

How to Remember Names

Do you remember the brand of the first refrigerator you ever had as an adult? What about the name of your wedding gown designer or the bank where you got your first checking account? Some people with exceptional autobiographical memory might. But if you don't, I bet you remember if the fridge didn't keep the ice cream cold, if the skirt of your dress went swish, or if the bank overcharged you for bounced checks. You'll likely remember the *essence* of those items, more than the *names* that went with them.

Same thing is true for people. Most people remember faces more than they remember names, so you can give yourself a break if you're one of the forgetters. But since many people do like it when you remember their names, here are some techniques that help you retain the "labels" of people you meet:

> **Notice.** Many people may not clearly hear the name of a new person the first time, especially since they don't care about that person—yet. Take a moment to be present to a new acquaintance's name.

> **Practice.** Say the name aloud to practice the motion of saying it. You can even just mouth it. Or ask for its spelling to reinforce both visual and auditory channels.

> **Use your senses.** Connect something you notice about the person to her name: "Loretta is wearing purple and drinking merlot at the bar." Again, say the name and the connection aloud to yourself to reinforce it.

> **Associate.** Connect the name to something familiar to use already active neural pathways. For example, associate the person with someone with the same name, such as your neighbor George with George Clooney. You'd think it would be confusing ("That's the sixth George I

know!"), but it helps. Or associate the new name with a familiar object. If you meet Harry Potter at a party, picture him with a big, hairy beard and turning clay on a wheel.

Link. Use your imagination and senses to make the name stand out. For John McCartney, you might think of pushing a big Port-a-Potty (John) in a cart (McCartney). Thinking of The Beatles would work, too!

Mnemonics

Mnemonic is a spelling bee word derived from the name of the Greek goddess of memory. A mnemonic is a memory aid; you connect what you want to know with something easier to remember: a rhyme, a phrase, funny images. I bet you know some mnemonics:

The Great Lakes: *HOMES*—Huron, Ontario, Michigan, Erie, and Superior.

The colors of the rainbow: *ROY G. BIV*—red, orange, yellow, green, blue, indigo, and violet.

Students use mnemonics to help them memorize the bones of the body, stars of the galaxy, or the classifications from species to kingdoms. Mnemonics that associate historic dates with memorable phrases can help students remember those dates on an exam.

We "regular people" can use mnemonics to remember a routine series of tasks, like what we need to do to close up a store at night. If you have to empty the cash drawer, turn off the *open* sign, and lock the warehouse door, it's easier to remember *COW* (**c**ash drawer, **o**pen sign, **w**arehouse door) than all three tasks individually.

Mnemonics are handy for helping you remember shopping lists, too. Let's say you want to remember to buy peanut butter, eye makeup remover, and sweet potatoes at the grocery store. Your wonderful, imaginative mind will help you create connections—connections that are lasting, funny, or weird, and familiar to you. Here are a few suggestions to get your brain started:

Peg. Connect your items to something that already has an order, such as *123, ABC,* or the letters of a word or phrase.

123. Imagine a six-foot-tall number *1* just inside the grocery store, and it's smeared with peanut butter; the number *2* has a fringe of eyelashes on the top, and you have *3* flashing, neon sweet potatoes in your cart.

ABC. Think of peanut butter on an **a**pple, eye makeup on a **b**oy, and sweet potatoes in the **c**art.

Letters of a word. Match the items to the letters of a word. For instance, I could not remember the order of the streets near my workplace even though I'd been there for years. A-ha! I could remember Taylor, Hampton, and Rogers using the word *three* since the three streets start with *T, H, R*. I haven't forgotten those *three* street names since.

Create a phrase. Take the first letters of each word and use them as the basis of a phrase. The first letters of peanut butter, eye makeup remover, and sweet potatoes are *P, E,* and *S,* which can equate to, "Pink elephants sit."

Link: Link items to each other in a mini story. Imagine your daughter wearing neon blue eye shadow and smearing a jar of peanut butter on the sweet potatoes.

Change a song. Change the words to a familiar song to reflect what you need to remember. If you have to pay bills, call the vet, and take out the trash, try using the song "Do-Re-Mi" from *The Sound of Music:* "Bills, are what I want to pay. Vet, is who I need to call. Trash builds up, must take away . . ."

Associate. Let objects come alive. They can merge, eat, or crash into each other, dance together, hug, have sex, smell like garlic—whatever is visual, absurd, emotional, rude, sensational, funny, and ridiculous. For example, imagine a giant garbage bag of bills emptying itself onto your poor dog.[153]

360 Degrees of Learning

Memory is one thing, but learning puts it all together. Unfortunately, many U.S. schools have eliminated music, arts, and recess, wanting to focus only on "useful" learning. But they're cutting off the proverbial nose to spite the face. By eliminating the arts and playtime, they prevent children from becoming the best in reading, writing, and arithmetic.

Music training increases the working-memory load, says Nina Kraus, brain researcher at Northwestern University.[154] It improves the ability to think, can raise IQ scores, and improve memory capabilities outside of music.[155] (I bet you can remember the lyrics to The Beatles' "Yesterday" without having memorized it.)

Arts training also strengthens the brain, particularly its attention system, and that can improve thinking and intelligence, says Michael Posner, PhD, of the Institute of Neuroscience at the University of Oregon.[156] A neuro-educational summit at Johns Hopkins University found tight correlations between arts training and improvements in cognition, attention, and learning.[157]

Play is also linked to attention. By playing, kids learn to wait for others, figure out what they want, ask questions, cooperate, imagine, try on roles (from president to mommy), and negotiate who plays what first. They develop executive functioning skills—the ability to organize thoughts, process information reasonably, hold relevant details in short-term memory, avoid distractions, and focus on the task at hand.

"Real playing is how real learning takes place," says visionary Joseph Chilton Pearce, author of *The Biology of Transcendence*. When playing, children are completely absorbed in their environment, building their knowledge of work, themselves, and the relationship between the two. "Play is the only way the highest intelligence of humankind can unfold."

Will play help adults learn? That's a new field of inquiry, but Stuart Brown, MD, coauthor of *Play: How It Shapes the Brain, Opens the Imagination, and Invigorates the Soul* and founder of the National Institute for Play, says that play is a profound biological process. Active play, by stimulating production of BDNF in the amygdala and prefrontal cortex, stimulates nerve growth for emotions and executive decisions.[158] The more that animals play, the larger their prefrontal cortices are.[159] Play also supports creativity by opening the mind, stripping away rules, and allowing unexpected connections to bloom.

Everyone knows how to play—or do they? Some types of play described by the National Institute for Play might expand your perspective and help you find new ways to play:

> **Attunement play.** Babies attune to caregivers through eye contact and baby talk. Adults can attune to others via improvisational theater or partner dancing. Sex works, too.

> **Imaginative, creative, and pretend play.** People usually save this type for Halloween, but you can play this way anytime by going wild with an air guitar, building an original Lego structure, or trying on personas in a costume store or a clothing department you rarely visit.

> **Body play and movement.** Sports are what most adults consider play. But diving into a lake or a pile of leaves, free dancing (sometimes called ecstatic dancing), or improvisational theater also qualify.

Storytelling/narrative play. At a family gathering or dinner, describe your day, when you got engaged, or your tenth birthday party. Or take a storytelling class.

Object play. Raid a toy store, practice juggling, rev up a race car, or get some Cubes—posable plastic managers and workers that can be placed in miniature plastic cubicles.

Social play. When your city sports team wins a championship, the whole sports-loving community plays and celebrates together. You can also wrestle, play board games, and have "parallel play," which is when you and a companion, while touring the zoo or a museum together, each go off on your own then come back together.[160]

But do you really have time to play, when there are so many other things on your to-do lists? Nina Wise, author of *A Big New Free Happy Unusual Life: Self Expression and Spiritual Practice for Those Who Have Time for Neither* understands this dilemma. Her book offers short, one- to ten-minute ways to express yourself in song, dance, poetry, and visual art.

Many of her students, she says, have felt that something was missing from their lives: "This gnawing in the heart is a longing to rekindle daily life with the spirit of self-expression, spontaneity, and play." Her activities open the door for you to be with yourself and the world in a whole new way.

Play utilizes your whole brain for learning. Here are some other ways for your whole brain to learn and remember:

Write. Jot a list of what you want to remember, keep a diary, or free write, in which you write without stopping for fifteen to thirty minutes. Continual writing helps you break through resistance or clarify where you need to go in your next steps. And go for a pen and paper, if you can. Experiments show that writing by hand triggers activity in significantly different portions of the brain than writing at a computer does.[161]

Enjoy music. Sing what you want to remember. Hum as you study. Play an instrument to stimulate different parts of your brain. Einstein played the violin to help him expand his thinking.

Move both sides of the body. Swing your arms as you walk. Stretch, sway from side to side, touch your right elbow to the left knee and vice versa a few times, or place your hands on opposite shoulders. (The last two are suggestions from energy medicine teacher Donna Eden.)

Play word games or do word puzzles. Play a game like Boggle, or do a crossword puzzle. Word (versus number) puzzles go beyond logic to help you visualize the objects or actions you come up with.

Juggle. This is great for concentration, and it also brings in play.

More on the Senses and Learning

There are three different ways of learning, based on what senses are primarily used: visual, auditory, and kinesthetic (through movement). Your preferred way of learning may show through your gestures and words. A visual learner might point as she talks about envisioning the future; an auditory learner tends to tilt her head to one side to listen better and mention that something resonates with her; a kinesthetic learner might touch your arm and talk about moving through a problem.

If you want to stretch your brain beyond how you usually learn, try doing a behavior from a different style. For instance, to enhance your visual-learning capability, look closely at the shades of colors in a painting or on a leaf, or pack the car trunk full of bags when you leave on a trip. You can increase your auditory-learning ability by singing, listening for the different instruments in a song, or imagining how an ocean wave sounds from beginning to end. To boost your kinesthetic-learning skills, massage your hands (or heck, get a massage) or notice how your gut feels when you make a decision.

Learning brings in the "light" of information through sight, sound, and feeling. Intelligence is where you aim that beam of light, or where your brain lights up naturally.

Are You More Intelligent Than You Realize?

Howard Gardner was one of the first to propose that humans had a wider variety of intelligences than that which was measured in the IQ test. As a professor of cognition and education at the Harvard Graduate School of Education, he based his theory of multiple intelligences on verification of particular types of intelligence in the brain and evidence that individuals existed with exceptional talent in these areas. "We all have all these intelligences," he says, although each person has them to varying degrees.[162]

The types of intelligence Gardner has identified are:

Linguistic: the ability to easily write, read, tell stories, and use language.

Logical-mathematical: fluency with numbers, logic, and reasoning. (This type is used in a broad range of tasks, from computer work to knitting.)

Musical: natural music talent, including identifying and using sounds, rhythms, pitch, and structures of songs.

Spatial: an expert sense of direction, hand-eye coordination, and visual memory.

Body-kinesthetic: dexterity and the ability to move well. (Carpenters, athletes, actors, and surgeons usually have this type.)

Naturalistic: a green thumb or feeling at home in the outdoors.

Interpersonal: the ability to lead, get along well with, and communicate with others; an awareness of others' moods and motivations.

Intrapersonal: the ability to focus on the inner person; self-awareness, recognizing one's goals and emotions.

Existential: "the intelligence of big questions" about life, death, infinity, and other dimensions. (Gardner is still exploring the validity of this intelligence.)

Technology buries us with information, as you'll see in chapter 10, but you can use it to help track the multitude of items you need to remember.

> **Calendars.** Set up appointments and reminders in calendars from Gmail, Outlook, cell phones, and other programs. They can remind you of an event with an email or text message, and they can even invite your son to the dentist and put the appointment on his electronic calendar. Or use calendars to remind yourself to send your sister her favorite birthday gift.
>
> **Tasks.** Programs can track due dates, completion, and priorities.
>
> **Information storage.** Programs can scan medical receipts, copy notes, read text—everything but call the bank and complain if there's an error.

Some programs, such as Evernote, Remember the Milk, Nozbe, and Toodledo, can link your computer to your smart phone. Cozi is organized especially for a family's busy schedule. Check reviews and top-ten lists before you jump whole hog into a program.[163]

Creativity

Do you enjoy making a great meal, arranging furniture, being funny, or even writing a nice card? When you do any of these things, you are being creative. Creativity is often defined as the ability to generate ideas, alternatives, and possibilities.

A few decades ago, when brain research was in its pioneer stages, scientists thought each part of the brain had one task. Word was that the right hemisphere was responsible for creativity, while the left one was in charge of organization and structure. In truth, both sides and the whole brain are involved in creativity, through a process called association.

When you're open to creative ideas, the first thing your brain does is check for existing or obvious solutions. The left hemisphere scans for remote, vaguely relevant memories—that's divergent thinking. Meanwhile, the right hemisphere searches for unseen patterns, alternative meanings, and high-level abstractions—that's convergent thinking. The associative cortex combines these abilities to lock onto an idea that works.

A note on the associative cortex: you use it in everyday life. It integrates information from your senses to let you know where you are in space. It also links emotions, logic, social abilities, language, skills, memories, movement, and thoughts to communicate in potentially novel ways, says Dr. Nancy Andreasen in *The Creating Brain*.[164]

You can expand your creative ability just by engaging it in different ways.

Ask questions. Preschoolers prime their creativity by asking "why, why, why?" Explore a few questions yourself: What instruments are played in the song that's on the radio? How would you redesign your house if money were no object? Why does your office have to handle every bill three times?

Take risks. I'm not talking about jumping a motorcycle over the Snake River Canyon, but push yourself to go a little out of the ordinary. Wear a reddish scarf with a lavender shirt. Tweet your favorite book. Add some red peppers to your lemonade.

Embrace failure. That's how you learn. As Thomas Edison said, "I have not failed. I've just found 10,000 ways that won't work." "Embrace failure" is another way of saying be kind to yourself.

Move. From walking to vigorous dancing, exercise spurs creativity, says Dr. John Ratey, author of *Spark: The Revolutionary New Science of Exercise and the Brain*.

Turn off electronic distractions. TV, the Internet, Facebook, solitaire, texting, books—they all engage just enough to seem useful, but they keep your brain from making connections. Let yourself get bored. Your brain will fill the idea void.

Practice your craft. Just do it, without trying to be creative or coming up with a new kind of birdhouse. Practice scales. Draw the same chair over and over. Why? Honing your skill increases your ability to manifest what you create. Having a pen in hand or buzz saw droning can also inspire creative visions.

Write. Writer and teacher Priscilla Long, author of *The Writer's Portable Mentor: A Guide to Art, Craft, and the Writing Life,* suggests that any artist do fifteen minutes of continuous writing to keep connected with their work. Write by hand, if you can. As Norman Mailer said, "It's hard to explain how agreeable it is to do one's writing in longhand. You feel that all of your body and some of your spirit has come down to your fingertips."

Play. You can view any task, even formatting a Visio document, through the lens of play.

Make creativity a habit. Put time on your calendar to do your art every day or every week. Make a creativity date, says Julia Cameron in *The Artist's Way,* to go to a museum, gallery, bookstore, or live performance.

Laugh. When you laugh, you're making connections between two disconnected items, which is just what you do when you're creative. Maybe George Carlin, Lily Tomlin, or Chris Rock will inspire you.

In addition to math, Renna used sensory stimulation to reignite her brain after her car accident. She spent time cooking and baking, and she started knitting. While all three activities involved math, they also engaged her brain with colors, textures, and smells.

Renna also used creativity to get her brain back in gear after her car collision. "Creativity was crucial! I researched the history of numbers, but more important, I think, was tactile creativity. That took the form of doll-making, which came out of nowhere: I did 3-D construction, sewing, embroidery, all kinds of creative problem-solving."

All of Renna's work stretched her whiplashed brain back into shape. She got her memory back, though her brain was different than it was before; her responses had more thoughtfulness and wisdom than previous spur-of-the-moment reactions.

You can make your brain different, too. Use the gifts you have—imagination, senses, learning, intelligence, association, and creativity—to engage with what's important. Your brain will be agile and happy, and so will you.

Chapter 7

Minding What Matters
How Thoughts, Emotions,
and Consciousness Affect the Brain

The pain of the mind is worse than the pain of the body.

Publilius Syrus, Roman author, first century BCE

If a cluttered desk is the sign of a cluttered mind,
what is the significance of a clean desk?

Laurence J. Peter, educator and author

Beth's brain knew she didn't have lice, but her mind didn't believe it. After she treated her son's head, immaculately cleaned her house, and got an all clear on her own scalp from a lice-experienced friend, she thought she could relax. But every little tingle on her scalp put her in a spiral of fear. She'd examine her fingernails after each head scratch, inspect the pillow case, and check all the possible symptoms on the Internet.

Funny, she thought, her head didn't bother her before her son got lice. Neither did her mind, and now they were in cahoots to drive her crazy.

Beth couldn't get her body and mind to go anywhere else.

Even without fear of lice, body and mind do not operate separately. Want proof? Consider a study in which a mirror was used to treat pain from amputations.[165]

Most amputees experience pain in their phantom limb; it's often from the sensation of ongoing clenching that the amputee can't release. V. S. Ramachandran, director of the Center for Brain and

Cognition at the University of California, San Diego, used a mirror box to help the *mind* release the *body's* pain. The mirror box hid the amputated limb while reflecting the image of the amputee's normal limb in its place.[166] When amputees were asked to relax or move both limbs, it looked to them like the phantom limb also relaxed or moved. The clenching pain ceased. Why? The mind saw evidence of the limb relaxing, even though the limb wasn't really there. Then the brain and body responded to what the mind saw.

You can't separate the body and mind, and you can't separate the body and the brain. All aspects of your interconnected system work together.

The Body-Mind in Action

What is the body-mind? You'll find many definitions that say it's "a connection between one's physical health and the state of one's mind or spirit." But that's just one aspect of the body-mind. Psychologist Alfred Adler said back in 1933, "Body and mind are co-operating as indivisible parts of one whole."[167]

The *body* part of the whole is clear you feel it, see your face in the mirror or your hand holding the book, and drive your body to work. The body is a noun, a thing.

The *mind* is not so easy to define. Merriam Webster says it's "the element in an individual that feels, perceives, thinks, wills, and especially reasons."[168] But you can't touch, see, smell, or hear that element because it's not a material organ. No matter how many biopsies of the body and brain you do, you won't find the mind. While the *mind* is a noun—a thing composed of thoughts, feelings, focus, perceptions, or judgments—it makes more sense to consider the mind to be the actions of verbs: *thinking, feeling, focusing, perceiving,* and *judging.* Your mind is always moving, always changing.

These thinking-feeling-action processes of the mind do live in a specific place: your body. The body needs the mind's mental processes to function, and the mind and brain need the body to act on thoughts and feelings. The body and mind go hand-in-hand (as it were).

*Your body needs the mind's mental processes to function,
and your mind and brain need the body
to act on thoughts and feelings.*

Knowing that the body and mind are one unit helps you influence the connections between your mind and body. This awareness provides you with more options, which change your experience of life. And then the brain creates new neural connections. This chapter highlights areas of body-mind connection where you can make a difference.

Your Abdominal Brain

Your gut—your intestines—contains more nerve endings than your brain does. Is this abdominal brain smarter than the one behind your eyes? Actually, they work together. The brain in your head interacts with the world, and the abdominal brain interprets the world and creates your perception of it.

Hey, Body, I'm Here!

Stimulus for the mind is all around—Internet, smart phones, Wii, email, Spider solitaire, Netflix, *The Sopranos* reruns. Even on a run around the lake, we pay attention to the iPod tunes. We live in a culture that makes it easy to ignore the body, to numb our physical sensations with activity, consumption, and entertainment. Not paying attention means we zone out (we're not all there), burn out (we experience illness or breakdowns), or lose out (we miss the joy of feeling our child's little hand in our own).

But even when our minds are full, our bodies are always still there, waiting for a little awareness.

"Paying attention to the body sharpens intuition, increases mental acuity and quickness, and expands our capacity to perceive through all of our senses," says Molly Gordon, business/life coach and owner of Shaboom, Inc. "It can even help break longstanding habits."[169] Paying attention to your body expands your brain and can make life bigger and brighter.

While it *seems* simple to be aware of the body, some overworked minds could use a little guidance. "Paying attention begins with being curious about the signs and signals your body sends," says Gordon. "Instead of shutting out sensations, explore them."

Here are a few ways to love your brain by noticing your body:

Explore one sensation. Close your eyes to reduce distractions. Notice a particular sensation in your body and how it feels. You may call the sensation *tension, relaxation, pain, numbness,* or *excitement,* but beyond that, what's the actual experience? Where is it located? How far does it spread? What is its temperature? Is there a texture, throbbing, expansiveness, or vibration to it? Ask yourself if there's any other sensory experience, like color or sound, that you associate with the sensation. Perhaps pain is purple or sounds like an electric saw, while joy is the color of yellow and sounds like a robin. Stay with the sensation in the body for a while. You will notice it change, fade, and maybe disappear for a little while.

Notice movement. Notice parts of your body as you move them: your fingers typing, your tongue licking your lips, your nose sniffling, your legs swinging as you walk, your lungs breathing in and out, your fingers turning the page, your hands and arms moving as you put groceries in the pantry or wash your hair in the shower.

Focus on your senses. Notice the feel of water when you wash your hands. Feel the heaviness of your bottom on the chair, or how your weight shifts when you're standing on one foot. Concentrate on the bass throb of music from a passing car or the whisper of your breath. Focus on the pattern in the movement of cars and busses on the street or the green clouds of leaves on trees. Take in the scent of the air after a rainstorm or the onions sautéing on the stove. Notice the tastes on different parts of your tongue when you eat and how tastes change as you chew and swallow.

Notice your sexuality. Pay attention to your body and ride the waves of excitement, focusing less on getting or giving an orgasm.

Notice your body's signals. Parts of your body—your tummy, eyes, jaw—can indicate your response to the environment and your thoughts. Your gut may clench when you enter a house overwhelmed with clutter, or when you know that a colleague's smile hides a mean streak. "Assume that the body knows something you don't," says Gordon, "and you'll be dazzled by its wisdom."

Emotions:
The Language of the Brain, Body, and Mind

In addition to physical sensations, the wisdom of the body comes through in another way: emotions.[170] "The vehicle that the mind and body use to communicate with each other is the chemistry of emotion," says Candace Pert, PhD, author of *Molecules of Emotion*. Emotions help you navigate life by:

- Allowing you to quickly get information about the surroundings,
- Enabling you to make decisions,
- Giving you feedback on how you perceive the world.

Emotions are also a global human language that help us connect with others. No matter where in the world you show anger, the natives will know what you're feeling. No translator needed.

"Brain science has begun to realize that the brain is not an organ of thought, but that it is a feeling organ that thinks," says Paul Mason, a neuroanthropologist (someone who studies culture and brain development).[171]

In fact, emotions, thoughts, actions, and sensations all happen at the same time, says Carrie Lafferty, physical therapist and Feldenkrais practitioner. Feldenkrais is a body-awareness program that helps make this interaction more visible.

We talked in the last chapter about how you remember exact details of an intensely emotional time, such as when you got married. Your whole limbic system gets engaged when you're experiencing a highly charged moment, which etches the experience in your brain. When scientists first studied emotions in the brain, they focused on the limbic system. The limbic system comprises brain structures bordering the inner surface of each cerebral hemisphere. It includes the hippocampus, amygdalae, thalamus, and hypothalamus. The limbic system is involved not only with emotions, but also motivation, sensory and sexual function, motor functions, and memory. (When we create a model of the brain with our two hands, as described in chapter 2, "Brain Basics," the limbic system is the imaginary ball of dough inside.)

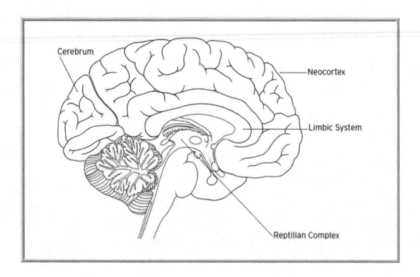

Emotion not only registers in the limbic system, but also echoes through the brain: in the prefrontal cortex (located in the front of the brain and managing planning, impulse control, emotional control, empathy, and more), in the anterior cingulate gyrus (which runs lengthwise through the frontal lobes and enables flexibility and adaptability to change), and temporal lobes (positioned beneath the temples and behind the eyes and controlling mood stability and sensory awareness).[172] Emotion changes your posture, facial expressions, heart rate, breathing, and awareness as it passes through your body.

Sometimes when a blast of anger, sadness, or self-hate hits you, you'd rather not have to deal those emotions. But avoiding emotions is not much of a life. Your emotions are what drive you to get up in the morning and go to work, lead you to form meaningful relationships, and help you make the right decisions for yourself.

Emotions are everywhere, but what are they exactly? And can changing your relationship to emotions affect the brain?

Some dictionaries define emotions as "subjective experiences involving both a mental state and a physiological state." That definition is a little too abstract. Others say emotions are a combination of thoughts, physical sensation, and the urge for action. But that combination could also describe hitting a baseball. What rides underneath those thoughts, sensations, and urges?

The definition that makes the most sense comes from neurolinguistic programming (NLP), a process that helps you replicate another person's behavior by first modeling that person's subjective (internal) experience. (For example, if you'd like to be more calm at work, you understand and mimic the language, body posture, and even thoughts of your coworker, so you too can focus on your paycheck instead of getting riled by the boss.)

In NLP, you pay attention to not just thoughts and emotions, but also how they're linked to create action. Emotions, according to NLP, are *meanings we associate with visceral sensations*—that is, how we interpret the responses of our abdominal brain and other central organs, such as our lungs, eyes, temperature, and heart rate. Those visceral responses arise from how we perceive things. Our emotions make us aware of what those perceptions are and, therefore, of how we experience life.

You might interpret a rapid heart rate, tightening of muscles, and sweating as signs of fear. Someone else could call them symptoms of excitement. Same physical responses, but two different perceptions of life experience.

Emotions come and go, arise and fall. If you're alive with a healthy brain, you will have a response—pleasant, unpleasant, and neutral—as you interact with the experience of life.

Emotions seem to tell you the truth. But do they really?

The Reality of Emotions and Their Triggers

Emotions feel real and 100% true. They include honest-to-God physical reactions.

And those reactions are accompanied by meaning: your series of thoughts that become your story of that part of your life. Your story creates a body response, so it's natural to assume that since the body response is genuine, the story must be just as true.

"Emotions are real," says Ragini Michaels, a spiritual teacher and author of *Unflappable: 6 Steps to Staying Happy, Centered, and Peaceful No Matter What.* "But they're not the whole truth."[173] They are verifiably true responses that you're having in your body, she explains, and absolutely true indicators of your perception of the world. But your perception is just one way of viewing the world. It is always valid, but never completely accurate, since it is only one of many possible points of view.

Recognizing Emotional Triggers

Let's say your hubby has dinner plans. In response to those plans, you might (1) look forward to having some downtime alone after work, (2) feel ignored by him, or (3) feel jealous of him for taking care of himself because you haven't created time for yourself.

Any of these reactions you have can be triggered or influenced by:

- The meaning or story you create about your life at the moment. For example, sometimes you feel delighted at a snow day; sometimes you're irate at the inconvenience it causes.

- A body response to which you ascribe a meaning. (Ever walk through the day ticked off, until you can find a "reason" for it, like stupid drivers in traffic?)
- Neurotransmitters such as serotonin, dopamine, and norepinephrine disorganized in the brain.
- Hormones—estrogen, progesterone, testosterone, oxytocin, steroids—rising and falling.
- Being around stressors and supporters.
- Illness and health.
- Exercise or the lack of it.
- Sleep and rest or the lack of them.
- The environment—nature or toxins.
- Healthy nutrition or the lack of it.
- The time of the year and the amount of natural light your body is getting. (Is the date closer to winter or summer solstice?)

Even though—actually *because*—there are many things that can trigger your emotions, you have a lot of resources for changing them, from taking vitamin D and using a light box to eating fish and reducing household toxins.

Dealing with Emotions

The physical sensation of uncomfortable emotions is, well, uncomfortable. Along with Beth's scratchy scalp, her stomach felt queasy with fear, and she resented feeling that way. These automatic reactions to emotions can create a muddle of despair, resentment, isolation, and more. On top of that, add the tendency to avoid painful emotions or sidestep them with addictions, repression, control, and/ or denial, and you often end up being controlled by your feelings.

"I think the fear of big, painful emotions is in not being able to see what's next," says advice columnist Carolyn Hax. "It's like when you're carsick, you can't imagine ever not feeling carsick." But several things help us change our relationship to emotions.

First is recognizing that emotions change. "Horrible feelings pass, the body can't sustain them," says Hax. "Even in the worst case, when somebody dies, the pain lessens with time—despite the fact that the loss remains constant."

Second, you see that life is naturally full of difficult emotions. Having them arise in your life doesn't mean you're bad, flawed, or manifesting incorrectly. There is summer (yay) and winter (bah); there is courage and fear, peace and anger, calm and anxiety. You can find lessons and balance while you're in the rotten, no good, horrible moods.

Third, you can lessen the intensity of, and your reactivity to, emotions by doing any of the following:

- Experience your emotions as they pass through your body. This helps you learn and get unstuck as you feel the sensations in your body. That may mean paying less attention to the story you create to notice the sensations.

- See a therapist to identify what you feel and find ways to express it.

- Do cognitive behavioral therapy to change your reactions.

- Talk to a friend to get a new perspective.

- Write. Spend ten minutes writing whatever streams through your consciousness to help you express your emotions and relieve the tension. Or write a nasty e-mail to express your feelings, but don't send it.

- Draw what you're feeling. Switch hands, or use both hands at once to access both sides of your brain.

- Sing and dance. There are some great sad country songs to wail, and your body can dance how happy, irritated, or blue you feel.

More ways abound to deal with emotions when you understand emotions are a *visceral response that you give a meaning to*. You can change the visceral response, change your meaning, or do both together (i.e., by using energy psychology, described below). Any of these changes helps you modify the intensity of emotions so they're not directing your life. The following ideas for diminishing the intensity of emotions can help you find what works for you.

Go slowly and monitor your comfort and reactions. While these suggestions work for many, be sure you have the support you need to create a change. A therapist can help you determine if these methods can work for you or suggest other paths.

To Change Your Visceral Response

Breathe:
- Gently exhale all the air from your lungs and let yourself naturally inhale.

- Do square breathing, where you keep the same count for all parts of the breath. For example, inhale as you count to four, hold the inhale as you count to four, exhale as you count to four, hold the exhale as you count to four, and repeat.

- Focus on three to ten breaths without doing anything else.

Relax:
- Tense and relax your muscles, starting with your toes and feet and progressing up to your face and scalp, or starting with your head and moving down.

- Simply relax your face—your eyes, cheeks, and lips.

- Loosen your jaw, both top and bottom, while feeling your head lighten up and drift back.

- Stretch, especially gently pulling back your arms and shoulders and opening your chest. (The chest is your center of love, including love for yourself.)

Connect with Nature: Walk outside. Buy a flower. Stand near a tree (or hug it, if you're of that ilk). Hang out at a beach. Water your plants. Notice how your existence is part of something bigger. (See chapter 13, "Beyond the Mind," for more on connecting with nature.)

Express Yourself: Write that nasty e-mail, then delete it. See a sad movie and cry. Laugh at yourself or at a funny movie. Yell into a pillow, allowing the sound and breath to come from deep in your belly. Go for a run and imagine stomping on what's bugging you.

See more in chapter 5, "The Dance of Your Body and Brain."

To Change Your Meaning or Perception

Rephrase Your Inner Talk: Listen to what you say to yourself and remind yourself of what's the bottom-line truth: you are a human who has reactions, makes mistakes, and is loving and alive.

Investigate Blame: Consider the saying, "When you point the finger of blame at someone else, you're pointing three fingers back at yourself." That means even though you're blaming someone else, what you're blaming him or her for are your own flaws. Applaud your courage to look at blame from a new perspective; it's not easy. Even if changing how you see blame doesn't resolve your hurt or anger, it can unearth empathy, which gives you more flexibility in your emotions and reactions. Byron Katie, author of *Loving What Is,* provides useful guidelines for this work of investigating blame.

Use Positive Talk: Positive talk can help you move away from a self-generating negative cycle. Thoughts, like emotions, naturally arise and fade. Some of them are negative, some of them are positive.

Eckhart Tolle, author of *The Power of Now,* says your thoughts are another form of perceptions and not the real you. You have the freedom to change your thoughts. You can also be aware of and counter thoughts that don't color the world the way you'd like. And you can *not* beat yourself up for thinking them.

Changing your thoughts can change your relationships to the emotions they bring up. If you're grumpy on Mondays, you can change the thought, "My boss drives me crazy" to, "I've got a job. Today I'll focus on the work, not him."

To Change Both Your Visceral Response and Meaning

Create: Creativity gives you a bigger view and can send the emotional energy out of your body. I know a woman who lost her family in an airplane crash; she transformed her grief into art by opening a store where people could make tiled memorial stones and benches.

Meditate: When you're quiet or focused on something else, you can diffuse the intensity of the emotional cycle rather than reacting to your emotion. Meditation gives you the chance to connect with something bigger than yourself and put the emotion into a broader context. (See chapter 13 for more on meditation.)

Use Energy Psychology: You can reduce emotional intensity by connecting with your electromagnetic field through various energy-psychology techniques. These techniques guide you to experience the emotion and change its intensity by changing the visceral response and meaning.

- Start by focusing on how the emotion feels in your body—in your head, chest, toes, and even sensations you might feel just outside of your body. The tips in the "Hey Body, I'm Here!" section of this chapter can help clarify what you feel.

- While doing the technique, focus on the emotion and make the physical sensations as strong as you can by bringing up scenarios that generate the emotion. Focusing on the emotion might sound scary, but doing so with kindness actually releases the emotion's intensity by short-circuiting its normal path through the brain and body. Then the emotional charge can move out of the body's energy field, leaving you feeling more calm and peaceful. Pay attention to how comfortable you are, and stop if the intensity is more than you can handle.

- In most cases, the physical sensations fade or feel more distant in five to twenty minutes. Check in with yourself to determine how long you need to do the technique.

When you're done with the technique, write down what you've learned and read it aloud.

> **Tapas Acupressure Technique (TAT)** is based on Traditional Chinese Medicine. Gently hold the bottom back of your head with one hand. Place the other hand so that the thumb and ring fingers hold spots on either side of the bridge of your nose—near the corners of your eyes; the middle finger touches the center of your forehead. As you let your sensations intensify, repeat phrases such as, "All the origins of this problem are healing now." Other phrases, such as those about blame and forgiveness, can also be helpful. (They are found on the Internet.)

Unwinding Frontal Occipital Holding is similar to TAT, but you gently hold one hand across your forehead and one hand at the back of your neck. Focus on your emotion, or just sit and let whatever's inside unwind.

Thought Field Therapy (developed by Roger Callahan) and the **Emotional Freedom Technique** (developed by Gary Craig) both involve tapping a series of points on your body while you repeat a phrase such as, "Even though I have this feeling of [whatever feeling you have, such as resentment], I fully and completely love and accept myself."

Begin by tapping the inner ends of your eyebrows. Then tap on the following points in this order: just outside the eyes, the cheekbones, just under your nose, under your mouth at the middle of your chin, under the inner collar bone, under your armpits where your bra goes, and on your liver (four to six inches beneath the right nipple).

If, after doing any of these techniques, the emotion and its accompanying sensation in your body don't fade, try this method, then do the energy psychology technique again.

Psychological Reversal Correction. Ever feel like you're going in circles or can't get your emotions and life aligned? Energy practitioners like Donna Eden suggest that your energy is going backwards. Psychological Reversal Correction adjusts your energy flow.

Follow your collarbone out about halfway toward the shoulders, then move two to three inches down until you find tender spots. Rub those spots and say aloud at least three times: "I completely accept myself with all my faults, problems, and limitations."

Then tap right under your nose and say aloud at least three times: "I completely accept myself, even if part of me is afraid I'll never get over this problem."

If your emotion is still stuck, you may need to pay attention to a different emotion first, or you might look for an energy psychology practitioner to help you out.

Move: Why is exercise listed under changing both your visceral sensation and the meaning you give it? Because exercise does both. Exercise expresses physical and emotional energy, and it creates a sense of accomplishment, which alters your attachment to emotional meaning and gives you a little distance from the drama of your story. Exercise also:

- Detoxifies your fight-or-flight stress response,
- Increases your endorphins, those natural feel-good hormones,
- Acts as an outlet for anger and hostility,
- Enhances your sense of personal strength and ability,
- Provides time for solitude or for a social connection,
- Deepens your breathing.[174]

A recent study at the University of Georgia found that exercise helps control emotions. Young men were monitored while watching disturbing slides. The following day, some of them exercised for thirty minutes while viewing the images again and others sat quietly while viewing them. The men who did not exercise had a higher level of anger.

Why? Scientists are not exactly sure, but one possibility is serotonin levels. Animal studies revealed that lower serotonin levels are associated with higher levels of anger. Lower serotonin levels are also believed to contribute to mood disorders in humans. And guess what increases serotonin levels? That's right—exercise. "Exercise for emotions is like taking aspirin to combat heart disease," said the study's lead researcher, Nathaniel Thom.[175]

If you read about exercise in chapter 5, "The Dance of Your Body and Brain," you'll discover how exercise affects the whole brain and new ideas on how to move.

You have opportunities for change when you feel stuck, because your body, brain, and mind are all interconnected; your body can change your mind, and your mind can change your body. For instance, you can imagine a flood of light unclogging your stuffed sinuses. You can remember all the things you're good at if you're feeling stupid as you learn to use new software. You can take a brisk walk if you have the blues when your son leaves for college.

Your interconnected being means you have opportunities for change and ways to see life from a new perspective—from right where you are now.

Chapter 8

Food

Take Your Brain Out to Dinner

Food is an important part of a balanced diet.

Fran Lebowitz, writer

Don't eat that! It's. . . too sweet, too artificial, too fatty, too fast, too processed, too fried, too salty, too carb-y, too cured, too glycemic, too meaty, too toxic, too weird, too wrong. . . . We have an obstacle course of food rules that we hope help us navigate the glut of foods surrounding us at the restaurant, grocery store, pantry, table, or from food carts on the street.

Most of those foods are processed. Almost half of Americans don't cook regularly, according to the American Time Use Survey from the Bureau of Labor Statistics.[176] So we let others do it, from restaurants to food-processing plants. That means we need food rules to make sure we eat what the body—not just the mouth—wants.

Processed foods are quick, for sure, but they often combine fat, sugar, and salt, and that triad makes you want more, according to David Kessler, author of *The End of Overeating.*[177] The food industry designs food to stimulate your brain, specifically the neurons that positively respond to certain tastes, textures, sights, smells, and temperatures. Those "palpable" foods trigger your opioid center, which releases chemicals (endorphins) that provide responses similar to those produced by heroin and morphine. Yep, food itself is addictive when it's made to be that way.

The food industry designs food to stimulate your brain, specifically the neurons that positively respond to certain tastes, textures, sights, smells, and temperatures.

Processing creates an adult baby food, Kessler says in his book—food that is easy to eat because the fiber, bran, and gristle have all been removed. This kind of food disappears quickly from your mouth after the first bite, which overrides the brain's feeling full signals.

While this chapter has suggestions on what to eat and what to avoid, you are the boss of your body, as they say in preschool. As you experiment with the new or stick with the familiar, notice what helps *your* brain to think better and keep your moods smooth. Then you'll have your own brain food, which is also good for the rest of your body.

The Skinny on Fats

We've had decades worth of advice about fats: eat vegetable oil, don't eat butter, eat margarine, don't eat trans fats, eat fish, don't eat margarine, eat butter. And recommendations are still shifting. But before we slather ourselves with fat, let's make sense of some of the terms.

Fats contain different kinds of molecules called *fatty acids.* Olive oil, corn oil, fish, animal products, and Hostess Twinkies all have various fatty acids. These fatty acids serve different purposes in the body. They may:

- Be burned for energy,
- Form structures for your cell membranes,
- Create steroids and cholesterol,
- Perform special duties in nerve cells and other tissues.[178]

The terms *saturated* and *unsaturated* fats (really fatty acids) refer to how the carbon and hydrogen are bonded in the molecule. And the bonds make a difference in how the fats are used in your body.

Saturated fats are straight chains of carbons all saturated or connected with hydrogen. One or more hydrogen atoms are missing from unsaturated fats, so the chain bends to bond to itself. *Monounsaturated fatty acids* have one double bond. *Polyunsaturated fatty acids* have two or more double bonds.

Your body and brain need some fats to function, but other fats can break apart in your body or throw the balance of fats out of whack.

Before news about fats became such a big deal, people ate mostly saturated fats, such as butter, meat fats, and even coconut and palm oil. Then during World War II, tropical saturated fats (coconut and palm oil) couldn't be shipped, and butter was rationed. Vegetable and seed oils came to the fore. They sounded good, since vegetables and seeds are nutritious.

Then in the 1950s, heart disease rose from a rare to a more common problem. Cholesterol was said to be the culprit, supposedly built up by saturated fats, which were starting to be used again. The agribusinesses and food industries that made vegetable oil supported that view. Whole businesses, from the drug industry to the diet industry, were developed around fighting cholesterol.[179]

But new studies show that the majority of people with high cholesterol never have heart attacks, said nutritionist Cherie Calbom in an article on fats for *PCC Sound Consumer*. If people do have heart attacks, saturated fats are probably not the cause. The Wynn Institute for Metabolic Research examined people who died of heart disease. Their plaques or clots were 26% saturated fat, while 74% was polyunsaturated fatty acids from vegetable oils and trans fats.[180] All of this information isn't encouraging you to pig out on lard and ignore cholesterol. Just know that cholesterol isn't the whole story. Some say that the increase in refined carbohydrates (white rice, white bread, white sugar) in our diets has more impact on heart disease than fats do.

But fats still matter to your health—and your brain.

Bad Fats

Damaged Fats—Find and Avoid Them: Fats can damage the body if they break apart, get rancid, have been heated beyond their capacity, or have been manipulated (as trans fats have been). Rancid and damaged fats can create *free radicals*, which cause a chain reaction of cell damage, and both the free radicals and fats can cause heart disease and cancer. These fats are being linked to inflammation, blood clots, and high blood pressure.

To avoid damaged fats:

- Throw out oils, nuts, and even whole wheat flour that smells rancid,
- Cook with oils at the right temperature,
- Keep oils in tinted glass bottles in a cool spot.

Still you may not notice other damaged oils, like those that have been manufactured using high heat, been treated to reduce rancid odors in packaged food, or been used to make trans fats. Avoid these by taking care in buying and eating prepared foods.

Trans Fats—Don't Eat Them: *Trans fats,* also known as hydrogenated or partially hydrogenated fats, are more stable, more solid, require less refrigeration, and spoil less quickly than other fats.[181] They're found in shortening, margarine, cookies, crackers, and snack foods.

Trans fats are made by taking the cheapest polyunsaturated oils, stirring in metal particles, and subjecting them to high-pressure and high-temperature hydrogen gas. Emulsifiers and starch are added to improve the consistency, and then the fat is steam-cleaned to remove the unpleasant smell. It can also be bleached to remove its lovely gray color, and artificial flavoring and coloring are added to make it more appealing.[182] Otherwise, no one would buy it.

Trans fats can keep your body from utilizing good, saturated and essential fatty acids. So your body uses trans fats to repair and develop cell membranes, which can lead to cell malfunction and a variety of health issues, including cancer, atherosclerosis, Alzheimer's, liver dysfunction, obesity, diabetes, immune dysfunction, birth defects, impaired vision, sterility, and weak bones and tendons.

Avoid trans fats by avoiding any food that lists "hydrogenated" or "partially hydrogenated" oil among its ingredients, even if the labeling says the product has 0 grams of either. Food is considered "trans fat free" if it has less than 0.5 gram of trans fat per itty-bitty serving. The American Heart Association allots only 1% of your total daily calories to trans fats—that's less than 2 grams a day.[183] A half of a bag of microwave popcorn contains about 5 grams. A single glazed doughnut can contain 3 to 4 grams. A McDonald's double Quarter Pounder with cheese has 2.5 grams.

If you love these foods, reduce eating them to maybe once a week, instead of once a day, or substitute other foods. If you like fast food, you can find menu items with little or no trans fats at Subway and Chipotle. Nutrition values for foods at various chains can be found online.

Polyunsaturated Fats—Mostly Not so Good: The molecule chain of polyunsaturated fats (PUFAs) is twisted and has more than one double bond. That means the fatty-molecule chains break easily and are more vulnerable to degeneration. Then these oils can cause free-radical damage, which has been implicated in heart disease and cancer. Too many polyunsaturated oils can also throw off the balance of good fats in your body, so you have more omega-6s than omega-3s (keep reading for information on these fatty acids). That imbalance increases inflammation, among other things, which is a precursor for heart disease.

To avoid PUFAs, eat less corn, soy, safflower, and sunflower oils (other than the high-heat ones below).

Good Fats—Increase Them

Saturated Fats—Useful in Moderation: Saturated fats (SUFAs) are good sources of energy and remain stable when they're cooked.[184] They come from animal products, like red meat, poultry, cheese, eggs, cream, and butter, as well as from tropical fruits, like palm fruits, palm kernals, and coconuts. According to Mary Enig and Sally Fallon in *The Truth About Saturated Fats,* these SUFAs:

- Give cell membranes necessary stiffness and integrity,
- Play a vital role in bone health by helping bones incorporate calcium,
- Protect the liver from alcohol and other toxins,
- Enhance the immune system,
- Help the body use and retain essential fatty acids,
- Become part of the fat around the heart, which the heart draws on in times of stress,

- Have important antimicrobial properties and protect the digestive tract against harmful microorganisms.[185]

Butter, a saturated fat, is much healthier than trans-fat margarine. Butter has vitamins A, E, K, and D. It can be used in medium-heat cooking; ghee (clarified butter, from which the protein has been removed) can be used for medium- to high-heat cooking. Avoid pollutants that cause cell damage by using organic butter.

Unprocessed, extra-virgin coconut and palm oil increase your metabolism, which raises your body temperature, boosts your energy and metabolic rate, and promotes weight loss. Use coconut oil for low- or medium-heat cooking and palm oil for higher-heat cooking.

Monounsaturated Fats—Good, but Be Careful With Cooking: These relatively stable fats are better than polyunsaturated fats, but less stable than saturated fats. They solidify in the fridge, but are liquid at room temperature.

Olive oil is great for salad dressings, cold foods, and low- or medium-heat cooking. To cook with higher heat, use avocado or almond oil. Canola oil can be used like olive oil, but nonorganic canola is likely to be genetically modified. High-heat or high-oleic safflower and sunflower oils are mostly monosaturated and can be used for cooking.

Omegas, the Essential Fatty Acids Your Body Loves: These are also PUFAs, but the good guys. Omega-3, -6, or -9 are named for where the double bonds are located in the (long) carbon chain. Of the three, omega-3s have been shown to be the most beneficial to both your body and brain. Omega-3s help with mood, cognition, disease prevention, and lots more.

Essential fatty acids are found in cold-water-fish, walnut, flaxseed, and certain vegetable oils. Specifically, you'll get omega-3s in fatty fish, as well as from soybean, corn, and safflower oils.

Think of omega-3s as the smartest, happiest, and most energetic of all the fats. When you lack omega-3s, your body will choose other fats instead, leaving you feeling grumpy and lethargic, with no energy left for thinking.

There are different types of omega-3s, but your brain really likes two: EPA (eicosapentaenoic acid) and DHA (docosahexaenoic acid). They're in fish, seafood, and algae. The other omega-3 is ALA (alpha-linolenic acid), which your body can convert, in small quantities (maybe 1 to 15%) to EPA and DHA. Flaxseed oil has high quantities of ALA, as do canola and soybean oils, chia seeds, and English walnuts.

Among their fabulous benefits, omega-3s

- Act as anti-inflammatories;
- Critically support brain and nerve development;
- Reduce the chance of a stroke;
- Lower blood pressure and cholesterol;
- Assist with attention deficit disorder (ADD);
- Reduce menstrual pain;
- Reduce the risk of colon cancer, prostate cancer, and possibly breast cancer and Alzheimer's;
- Support positive moods.

After reading all of this great information about omega fatty acids, you're likely to say, "Bring on the omegas!" But you need to be specific to get what your body and brain really want: only omega-3s and mostly the EPA and DHA omega-3 fatty acids.

What about omega-6s and omega-9s?

Omega-9s lower cholesterol levels, reduce atherosclerosis (hardening of the arteries), and improve blood-sugar levels and immune function.

Omega-6s increase or regulate blood clotting, cell proliferation, skin and hair growth, metabolism, the reproductive system, and inflammation. They can also help with rheumatoid arthritis, allergies, eczema, psoriasis, and rosacea. Sounds good, right? But these benefits come only when you have omega-6s in the right ratio with omega 3s; too many omega-6s can create inflammation inside your body.

You're likely already getting way *too many* omega-6s. You get omega-6s in meat (mostly as PUFAs), processed oils, and processed foods—mainly foods from grocery shelves and fast-food restaurants.

The ideal ratio is at least twice as much omega-3 as omega-6s (some say 4:1). The typical American ratio is about 1:14 to 1:25.

Time to up the omega-3s from fatty fish, like salmon, mackerel, herring, lake trout, sardines and albacore tuna—good sources according to the American Heart Association. However, there may be some downfalls to consuming a substantial amount of our swimming buddies.

Farmed salmon are widely known as being carriers of PCBs (polychlorinated biphenyls), which are industrial chlorine contaminants. Even though the manufacture of PCBs was banned in 1979, these chemicals still exist, and their affects are still being seen. A major 2003 study by the Environmental Working Group found that farmed salmon contained sixteen times the PCBs that wild salmon contained. [186] Recent studies show that levels of PCBs in farmed salmon are declining, but continue to remain higher than levels in wild salmon. Exposure to PCBs affects your brain's IQ, among other problematic responses.

You can instead take fish-oil supplements, looking for those from nontoxic fish. Get supplements with about 1,050 mg of EPA and 150 mg of DHA, and take them at bedtime. Keep them in the freezer if you get a fish-oil burp. *Don't* get supplements with omega-6 and -9; those omegas are the last thing you need.

How can vegetarians get their EPA and DHA? Microalgae oils are becoming popular, and while they provide plenty of DHA, they provide less EPA. Still, these oils are a good start.

Krill supplements are also the latest thing, but it's unclear if they are a viable substitute for fish-oil supplements. Krill are tiny, shrimplike creatures that live in huge numbers in polar seas. They are the main food of some whales, sharks, rays, seals, and seabirds. Krill oil should provide all the potential health benefits of fish oil, might have a longer shelf life, and doesn't give you the fish-oil burps. Krill oil is more expensive than fish oil. There are also environmental questions: Some say there are plenty of krill to spare, so consuming them is not a problem. Others are concerned that krill harvesting may destroy local krill bio-niches in the pristine waters of Antarctica. Keep your eye out for further studies.

Vegetables

If you're looking for a surefire way to slow cognitive decline, stock up on veggies. Not only do the antioxidants in vegetables protect against oxidation, but vegetables have also been linked to a delayed onset of Alzheimer's disease. One study showed that elderly folks who ate nearly three servings of veggies every day slowed their natural aging cognitive decline by 40%.[187] **Greens,** such as spinach, kale, and collards, help reduce natural cognitive aging. Older rats fed a large amount of spinach showed significantly improved learning and motor-skills capacity.[190] Spinach may lessen brain damage from strokes and disorders.

Sweet potatoes and other dark-colored veggies, like bok choy and watercress, are loaded with B-6, the antioxidant vitamin C, and beta-carotene. (For more on what these vitamins do for your brain, see the vitamins section at the end of this chapter.)

Cruciferous veggies (including cabbage, broccoli, and collard greens) have vitamins and indole-3-carinol, a chemical that repairs damaged DNA.

How many vegetables should you eat? The U.S. Department of Agriculture now suggests five to nine servings per day. Women ages nineteen to fifty should consume 2.5 cups of veggies per day, and women ages fifty-one and up should eat 2 cups. The men in your life (at least those ages nineteen to fifty) should eat 3 cups per day, while men fifty-one and up should eat 2.5 cups. (You don't have to cram lettuce into measuring cups. Just remember a cup is about the size of a fist or tennis ball.)

Women under the age of fifty should eat 2.5 cups of vegetables daily; women over fifty should eat 3 cups.

If you have a hard time adding veggies to your diet, try precut broccoli and sugar peas from the salad bar, baby carrots, or steaming frozen veggie combos. Keep your veggies in sight, washed and trimmed, so you don't end up with limp ones in the back of your fridge. Sneak them in other dishes like soup, which can handle pretty much any type of veggie you want. Drinking veggie juice is an easy way to add nutrients, but many dieticians encourage limiting juice intake to one serving per day, since it doesn't have the valuable fiber that whole veggies do.

Fruits

Though they don't replace veggies, fruits have lots of plusses for the brain. Fruits provide phenolics, chemicals that protect the brain from damage leading to Alzheimer's and Parkinson's disease, and flavonoids, a large class of plant pigments that are antioxidants and reduce neuro-inflammation and brain aging.[189]

Avocados are among WebMD's top five foods for promoting brain health. Not only are they full of fiber, vitamins, and potassium, but they also contribute to the prevention of breast, oral, and prostate cancer, as well as strokes. They are also credited with promoting eye and heart health, among other benefits.

Blueberries are famously awesome for your brain. They help memory, motor skills, balance, and coordination and are full of anti-oxidants. Blueberries help arteries contract—good for blood pressure. They even reduce the damage of a stroke from a blood clot. In a study, rats that ate a blueberry-enriched diet learned better than their non-blueberry-eating friends.[190]

Strawberries are also loaded with antioxidants and contain a chemical called fisetin, which has been shown to increase memory. Fisetin is also found in tomatoes, onions, oranges, apples, and kiwi.

Apples, especially red ones like Red Delicious and Northern Spy, contain brain-protecting phenolics. Put Fuji apples at the top of your list, since they have the highest totals of phenolic and flavonoid compounds.

Red grapes benefit brain cells and can improve cognitive function—even reverse aging of neurons, according to an article in *Nutrition Journal*.[191]

In a preliminary study, mice that were fed **pomegranate juice** raced through mazes 35% more quickly than their peers, indicating that the pomegranate juice increased learning and memory.[192] Pomegranate-fed mice also had 50% less Alzheimer's (plaque) buildup in the brain.

> ## Amazing Chia Seeds
>
> Chia seeds are tiny, but they pack a whole lot of nutrition. A pouch of chia seeds would sustain Mayan warriors and hunters if food was scarce. Chia is rich in omega-3s (the same ALA type that's in flax, some of which can be converted to more usable EPA and DHA), has six times the calcium contained in milk and three times the iron found in spinach, and puts goji and blueberries to shame for antioxidants. They also sprout green hair, creating those chia plant pets that used to be popular! How do you eat these little seeds? Sprinkle them on salads or cereal, add a quarter teaspoon into a milkshake, eat them ready-made in cereals and chips, or put a little into a large glass of water, where they turn into a good-for-you gel. They fill you up with good nutrition.[193] You can buy chia seeds in natural foods stores or online.

Spices

The chemical curcumin that turns **turmeric** yellow appears to activate an antioxidizing enzyme that reduces plaque buildup. It also is an anti–inflammatory that fights some cancers and multiple sclerosis.

Saffron fights depression and improves PMS symptoms by increasing serotonin levels in the brain. Saffron twice a day was as effective as Prozac in treating mild to moderate depression.[194] While saffron is expensive—eight to twelve dollars per gram—a few threads in your cooking (heat and liquid release its essence) might make you feel better at the end of dinner.

Sage, also known as garden meadow, helps guard against depletion of the neurotransmitter acetylcholine, which is crucial to proper brain function. You can add a bit of sage to salads, soups, and pizza.

Fresh sage adds a livelier taste and smell. Research continues on whether **ginkgo biloba, sage,** and **rosemary** prevent or slow the development of Alzheimer's disease.

Oregano is packed with antioxidants. In fact, you can get the same amount of antioxidants from a tablespoon of fresh oregano—or 1/2 teaspoon of dried oregano—as you do from an apple. For more about the benefits of antioxidants, see the antioxidants section at the end of the chapter.

Cinnamon boosts brain function, says the Agricultural Research Service, and triggers memory.[195] Chewing cinnamon gum enhances memory, visual-motor speed, recognition, attention, and focus. Cinnamon also helps regulate sugar levels; reduces proliferation of leukemia and lymphoma cancer cells; reduces clotting of blood platelets; acts as an antimicrobial, meaning it helps with yeast infections; contains the trace mineral manganese; and is a very good source of dietary fiber, iron, and calcium. Apples and cinnamon are a great snack—especially for kids doing homework.

Brain Beverages

Coffee and Caffeine

Recent statistics say that 50% of adult Americans drink coffee every day. That's roughly 150 million Americans drinking just over three nine-ounce servings per day. What does coffee do to our brains?

No surprise, it's the caffeine in coffee that has the most powerful impact. Caffeine has been shown to improve athletic performance as much as 70%. It is so powerful that the International Olympic Committee lists caffeine as a doping agent. Caffeine also protects your blood-brain barrier, a thin filter that protects your central nervous system from potentially harmful chemicals carried around in the bloodstream.[196] In recent studies, caffeine has been shown to improve the speed and accuracy of certain intellectual tasks, as well as help neurons form longer lasting connections; in short, it can improve your memory. Moderate use of caffeine can also help the brain respond more energetically to stimulation.

But all these perks come at a price. If you're a heavy coffee drinker, you can expect to feel lethargic during your afternoon caffeine rebound, says Dharma Singh Khalsa, MD, in his book *Brain Longevity*.[197] Too much caffeine can also lead to restlessness, rambling thoughts and speech, digestive upset, tremors and twitching, diureses (peeing lots of urine), and agitation. You might be willing to live with these effects, but too much caffeine may also cause panic attacks or anxiety. Experiment with drinking different amounts of coffee and/or caffeine to see what minimum amount gives you the benefits without the drawbacks.

If cutting back on caffeine is the right move, try mixing decaf coffee with regular coffee or drinking green tea, which has less caffeine. Or try a natural picker-upper like veggie juice or a piece of fruit, which give you a quick energy boost through a shot of fructose.

Green and Black Tea

Like coffee, green and black tea both contain caffeine. Black teas usually have half as much caffeine as coffee, and twice as much as green teas; white teas have a little less than green teas. But teas also have plenty of brain-boosting properties.

Tea protects brain cells from degeneration and keeps your mind sharp. Natural compounds in tea, called catechins, protect your brain cells from a buildup of protein that interferes with cognitive function. Catechins also provide nerve energy and may be anti-carcinogenic, anti-inflammatory, and antimicrobial (meaning they fight the growth of bacteria, viruses, and fungi).

And there's more. Polyphenols in tea support mood, provide antioxidants for the heart, protect against brain disorders and Parkinson's disease, and keep glucose levels (which affect brain-energy levels) steady. Tea's tannins help the brain recover from stroke and other brain injuries. They also stimulate the brain to create relaxing alpha waves—that's the same calm brain activity that occurs while you're resting with your eyes closed. The amino acid L-theanine, found almost exclusively in tea, may help your mood and learning by increasing serotonin, dopamine, and anxiety-reducing GABA (gamma-aminobutyric acid) levels.[198]

Green and black teas also protect against the destruction of certain neurotransmitters—the same way some drugs that treat Alzheimer's do. White tea (made from tea leaves that are picked earlier than green or black tea leaves, when the buds still have a fuzzy coating) may fight depression and protect nerve cells. The website WebMD suggests drinking two cups of tea per day.

Alcohol

On one hand, alcohol contributes to brain shrinkage. Individuals who had at least two drinks a day shrunk their brains an average of 1.6%. And women experienced greater alcohol-induced shrinkage.

On the other hand, you may have heard about the benefits of red wine. Do they offset the negative effects of alcohol? Resveratrol and flavonoids found in red grapes and wine can improve cognitive function. If you're healthy, not taking medicines that interact with alcohol, and are not addicted to alcohol, one glass of red wine per day (one to two glasses for men) can reduce the incidence of Alzheimer's disease. Grape juice and possibly dark beer have similar effects.

There is a fine line between what's good and what's bad for you with stronger alcohol. Light alcoholic drinking (one to four drinks a week) can reduce the risk of ischemic (clotting) strokes, while heavy drinking (three-plus per day) increases the risk of stroke by 45%, according to the Beth Israel Deaconess Medical Center.[199] Alcohol is a blood thinner, so check with your doctor if you're taking aspirin or other thinning agents, such as warfarin (Coumadin) or heparin.

Soda

Soda protects your body and brain from absolutely nothing, and it depletes your body of vitamin A, calcium, magnesium, and water—which you may remember are crucial for your brain. Minimizing or avoiding soda is a good strategy for taking care of your brain.

Water

The giant sponge in your skull is more than 78% water, and so you don't want to dry it out. Even a small drop in your drinking level can make your brain's performance drop 20 to 30%.

> *Not drinking enough water can decrease*
> *your brain's performance by 20 to 30%.*

Water keeps your brain hydrated. It also is a transportation service for the cells in your body, bringing in nutrients and carrying out waste products. If you become dehydrated, your cells begin clogging with waste and will eventually starve to death due to lack of nutrients.

The general guideline is 64 ounces of water per day, but it really depends on your body, the weather, and your activity level. Your urine will generally be pale when you're getting enough water. If you're not a water fan, don't worry. You can get much of your recommended intake from tea, fruits, and veggies. Packets of Crystal Light and Propel drink mixes can also make your water taste, well, not like water. But don't count soda, coffee, or alcohol as part of your water intake. Those are all diuretics, taking water away from your body and brain.

Other Foods and the Brain

Some other common foods that can affect your body and brain include the following.

Egg yolks contribute a fatty chemical called choline to your diet. Choline is responsible for brain health and function and can reduce the mental decline of aging and possibly the incidence of Alzheimer's disease.

Chocolate has the power to delay the decline of your brain and help boost your cognitive functions during challenging mental tasks, say scientists at the American Association for the Advancement of Science in San Francisco.[200] Flavanols, a naturally occurring nutrient in fresh cocoa, may be the source of chocolate's brain-boosting power.

The chemicals in the cacao/cocoa bean, from which chocolate is made, mimic the rush of falling in love and the altered state that comes from marijuana. But like coffee, chocolate is not without side effects. Too much chocolate can cause headaches, restlessness, insomnia, tachycardia (rapid heart beats), agitation, and anxiety. Some of these symptoms arrive with withdrawal—when the buzz is over. Just like with coffee, it might be wise to experiment with the amount of chocolate you nibble on to find out how much does you good without doing you harm.

Salt is a mineral that's probably best to minimize. Your taste buds love salt, but it can create high blood pressure for some people. So how to minimize salt in your diet? Cook more at home, use herbs and spices instead, and eat fewer premade foods.

Sugar and refined carbohydrates excite your taste buds—and brain—though your body has to produce insulin to balance them all out. After the sugar rush, there's too much insulin, and you may feel spacey, weak, or anxious. Sugar itself and high-fructose corn syrup (found in more foods than you'd think, including salad dressings, lunch meat, and crackers) can also lead to diabetes, which sets the stage for stroke. Look for sweeteners that include beneficial nutrients, enzymes, and antioxidants, such as raw honey, real maple syrup, and sucanat.

Artificial sweeteners have the blessing of the U.S. Food and Drug Administration, although other organizations, such as the National Cancer Institute, have major concerns about them. To avoid them, some folks go for fruit-juice sweetener, Stevia (made from a plant leaf), and maple syrup. Agave nectar (which comes from a dessert succulent), and Truvia (a combination of Stevia and the sugar alcohols xylitol and erythritol) are touted as natural, but are generally highly processed. Agave nectar may have a considerably higher fructose concentration than high-fructose corn syrup, and fructose is processed by your liver rather than your digestive system.

Antioxidants

Antioxidants reduce the effect of oxidation in your brain cells when old neurons age and die. *Oxidation* is a crucial chemical reaction (think of a cut apple turning brown) that forms *free radicals*. Free radicals can be beneficial to your metabolism and help your immune system fight viruses and bacteria, but they can also start chain reactions that damage cells. Free radicals are basically atom bonds that are unstable because they are missing electrons. So they try and capture electrons from other compounds to gain stability. When they steal electrons from nearby molecules, they turn those molecules into unstable free radicals. This chain reaction can get out of control, altering DNA, mutating cell membranes, and causing cell death.

Protect your neurons by getting plenty of antioxidants in your diet. The Mayo Clinic suggests that you eat a wide variety of high-antioxidant foods (instead of focusing on just one), such as:

Berries—blueberries, blackberries, raspberries, strawberries, and cranberries,

Beans—small red beans and kidney, pinto, and black beans,

Fruits—apples (with peel) such as Red Delicious, Granny Smith, and Gala; avocados; cherries; green and red pears; fresh or dried plums; pineapples; pomegranates; and kiwis.

Vegetables—artichokes, spinach, red cabbage, red and white potatoes (with peel), sweet potatoes, and broccoli,

Beverages—green tea, coffee, red wine, and many fruit juices, such as pomegranate,

Nuts—walnuts, pistachios, pecans, hazelnuts, and almonds,

Herbs—ground cloves, cinnamon, ginger, dried oregano leaf, and turmeric powder,

Grains—oats

Dark chocolate (it ranks as high or higher than most fruits and vegetables for antioxidant content).[201]

As a bonus, many foods high in antioxidants typically offer many other health benefits, such as high fiber, protein, and vitamin and mineral content, and they are low in saturated fat and cholesterol.

Vitamins

Your brain needs vitamins to communicate, protect, and clean itself; to stay as young and healthy as possible; and especially to protect itself from damaging free radicals. You can also get antioxidants and other good stuff from vitamin supplements. If you have questions about supplements, check a reliable source, such as the University of Maryland Medical Center's online Medical Alternative Medicine Index, the Bastyr Center for Natural Health website, or Dr. Andrew Weil's website. The following recommendations come from one of these sources. (See the resources list in the back of the book for the website addresses.)

Vitamin D is the "in" supplement for good reason: it promotes bone health, regulates calcium levels, and may reduce the risk of multiple sclerosis, cardiovascular disease, and even diabetes, according to the Harvard School of Public Health.[203] And it helps your brain. While scientists are in early research stages, they know that vitamin D regulates brain enzymes, helps you synthesize neurotransmitters, helps grow and protect neurons, and reduces inflammation. On top of that, two large studies showed that lower vitamin D levels lead to significantly lower cognitive function. Studies are planned to see if it helps reduce the risk of Alzheimer's in healthy older adults.[204]

Naturopath Eileen Stretch says that if people could only take two supplements, she'd suggest fish oil and vitamin D.[205] How much vitamin D do you need? It depends on your skin color, where you live, and how much you get out in the sun, but experts suggest 1,000 to 2,000 IU daily—about what you'd get if you were in the sun for fifteen to thirty minutes a few times a week.

The **B vitamins** help your brain with energy, nerve connections, and nerve health. Thiamin (vitamin B-1) converts food (carbohydrates) into fuel (glucose), which is the brain's primary energy source. It synthesizes neurotransmitters and, together with the rest of the B vitamins, helps the nervous system function. An anti-stress vitamin, thiamin may also strengthen the immune system. It's in whole grains, pork, legumes, nuts, seeds, and organ meats. Supplements if desired: 50 mg as part of a B-complex supplement.

Vitamin B-12 maintains the nerve cell's outer coating, preventing nerve damage and impaired brain function such as dementia and brain atrophy. B-12 works closely with vitamin B-9 (folate) to help the functions described below. Animal foods, such as milk, meat, and eggs, have B-12, as do some fortified cereals, nutritional or brewer's yeast (inactive yeast that's rich in protein, vitamins, and minerals—and pretty tasty on popcorn), and soymilks. Supplements if desired: 50 mcg as part of a B-complex supplement.

Note that about half the soy crop has been genetically modified, with controversy about who is funding the research of their safety. If you're concerned, look for "non-GMO" on the labels of soy, milk, and other foods you buy.

Folic acid or folate (B-9) is crucial for proper brain function—especially in conjunction with B-12. Folate is the nutrient most largely associated with depression. Folate increases cognitive function, but it has not yet been proven to reduce the risk of Alzheimer's disease. Pregnant woman take folate to reduce neural-tube defects in their babies.

And while not directly affecting the brain, higher folate intake is associated with a reduced risk of breast cancer and is related to proper DNA replication and repair. To boost your folate levels, add spinach, turnip greens, romaine lettuce, liver, nutritional yeast, asparagus, dried beans and peas, wheat, broccoli, and some nuts to your menus. Supplements if desired: 400 mcg per day as part of a B-complex supplement.

Vitamin B-6 is essential for the production of most of the brain's neurotransmitters. Along with B-12 and folate, B-6 helps you process the S-adenosylmethionine (SAMe) your body produces. (You might take SAMe as a supplement.) Without SAMe, you're more likely to have depression, dementia, or nerve degeneration. B-6 is found in chicken, fish, pork, whole wheat products, brown rice, and some fruits and vegetables. Supplements if desired: 50 mg per day as part of a B-complex supplement.

Vitamin C is an essential antioxidant we get from citrus fruits, parsley, bell peppers, strawberries, papaya, and cruciferous veggies (such as broccoli, cauliflower, kale, mustard greens, and brussels sprouts). Vitamin C helps synthesize the neurotransmitters, including serotonin, dopamine, and norepinephrine, which you need to have healthy brain function and moods. With vitamin C, your body can synthesize the amino acid carnitine, to transport fat for brain energy. Vitamin C also recycles other antioxidants such as vitamin E, restoring their power after use, and helps produce collagen for blood vessels. Supplements if desired: 250 mg of vitamin C each day.

Vitamin E is an antioxidant that readily enters the brain. Its ability to help prevent Alzheimer's disease hasn't been proven, but it may improve cognitive function for those who are healthy or have non–Alzheimer's dementia (for example, those who've had several strokes). However, it's clear that excessive vitamin E supplements do not benefit your health. You can get vitamin E from wheat germ, vegetable oils, nuts, avocados, green leafy vegetables, and fortified cereals. Supplements if desired: 400 to 800 IU daily of a product with mixed natural tocopherols.

Minerals

Minerals are a hidden treasure; most of us don't realize their benefits. Even in trace amounts, they provide for electrochemical nerve
activity, maintain delicate cellular-fluid balance, form bone and blood
cells, and regulate muscle tone and activity. Many are antioxidants and
are used for all enzyme activities.

Boron is a trace mineral with a critical role as a coenzyme (a
small molecule that assists the functioning of an enzyme) in chemical
reactions. Boron increases cognitive ability, says the National Institutes of Health.[206] It also strengthens the immune system, increases
the amount of calcium that is absorbed from food, boosts energy
utilization, and positively affects cholesterol production. Some
reports say that boron increases memory and hand-eye coordination, as well as easing arthritis, fatigue, migraine headaches, nervousness, depression, and osteoporosis. You'll find boron in fruit, such
as pears, apples, peaches, grapes, and raisins; nuts and peanuts; leafy

veggies; and beans. If you take supplements, the recommended dosage is 3 mg per day.[207]

Iron is essential to the formation of hemoglobin, which carries oxygen for the brain's energy process. Without enough iron, you may be slowed by anemia, the most common blood condition in the United States, affecting about 3.5 million Americans. Women and those with chronic diseases have an increased risk of anemia, so make sure to stock up on iron-rich foods, like meat, poultry, and fish. Iron can also be found in whole grains, green leafy vegetables, dried beans and peas, and dried fruits. Using a cast iron frying pan is another great way to get your iron.

Iron supplements are usually given to those with iron-deficiency anemia, and they can cause serious constipation. Liquid supplements, chewable ones (may stain some teeth), or slow-release iron are more digestible; taking them *with* vitamin C helps with their absorption, but *do not* take iron supplements with calcium. Check with your doctor for the right dosage.

Magnesium is a fabulous mineral for your brain, as it helps transmit nerve impulses. A deficiency creates nervousness and twitching. Magnesium also supports bone health and can help prevent migraines. You'll find magnesium in green leafy vegetables, firm tofu, halibut, potato skins, whole grains, nuts, seeds, bananas, and—yes indeed—chocolate. Supplements for adult women are 250 to 300 mg daily, but too much leads to soft stools and/or diarrhea.

Manganese is a trace mineral that also contributes strongly to brain function. Low levels of manganese can contribute to infertility, bone malformation, weakness, and seizures. Avoid these conditions by eating plenty of nuts and whole grains (refined grains provide only half as much manganese as whole grains do). The amount of manganese ingested in one day (from foods or supplements) should not exceed 10 mg due to the potential for nervous system damage.

Copper, along with iron, maintains the brain's biochemistry. Copper helps with proper growth and benefits your hair, eyes, and energy production. Copper deficiency, on the other hand, impairs brain and immune system functions, changing certain chemical receptors in the brain and lowering neurotransmitter levels. And it also has some pretty serious symptoms, including anemia, low body temperature, and elevated cholesterol levels. The best way to get copper is by eating organ meats, seafood, nuts, seeds, whole grain breads and cereals, and chocolate. If you take a supplement, the recommended daily intake is 900 mcg, but you should also take zinc supplements (8 to 15 mg of zinc for every 1 mg of copper), since an imbalance of these two minerals can cause other health conditions.[208]

Zinc protects against neural disorders and is an antioxidant. It maintains cell membranes and protects cells from damage, supports proper immune-system function, reduces stress, improves metabolism, and supports the healing of acne and wounds. Zinc deficiency can create neurological problems, sensory impairment, and reactions ranging from apathy and fatigue to irritability and jitteriness. Zinc is found in red meats, liver, eggs, dairy products, vegetables, and some seafood. Most people get 10 to 15 mg from food per day.

Zinc sulfate, a common form of zinc found in supplements, can cause digestive problems. Other types of zinc include zinc citrate, zinc picolinate, zinc acetate, zinc glycerate, and zinc monomethionine. Women should get around 8 mg per day, according to the U.S. recommended dietary allowances. Therapeutic doses can range from 35 to 45 mg, but check with your doctor if you take more than 40 mg, and if you take high doses for more than a few days.[209]

Selenium may regulate your cognitive function. Selenium also helps synthesize certain hormones and protect cell membranes from damage, and it is possibly beneficial in cancer prevention. This trace element can be found in nuts, liver, seafood, and eggs. Do not take supplemental selenium without checking with your doctor, since it can increase your risk of getting diabetes. You should not need to take extra selenium unless you smoke, drink alcohol, take birth-control pills, or have a digestive malabsorption syndrome, such as Crohn's disease or ulcerative colitis.

$\mathcal{C}\!\sim$

Do you need an expensive trip to the supplement store to get your vitamins and minerals? While a multivitamin can't hurt, if you stick with a healthy, balanced diet, you won't need to supplement with expensive pills. Plus, real food—especially veggies and fruits—offers more benefits than just vitamins and minerals.

If you do decide you need dietary supplements, let your health care provider know, because they might have side effects or interactions with medications.

Enjoy Your Food!

No matter what you eat, enjoy it! Food sustains your body, eases your hunger, and creates community, and everything about it—its color, smell, texture, crunch, and taste (from tart to sweet)—can stimulate all five senses.

The experience of food is good for your brain.

Chapter 9

The Brain and the Environment
Toxins-Schmoxins

*Not all chemicals are bad. Without chemicals
such as hydrogen and oxygen, for example, there would be
no way to make water, a vital ingredient in beer.*

Dave Barry, humorist

When she learned she had cancer, Fran Drescher took a new look
at her facial cleanser. The star of the TV comedy *The Nanny* wasn't
concerned about her skin. She just didn't want to be pouring toxins
on her face—or anywhere else on her body.

Drescher found there was more to beating cancer than surgery,
chemotherapy, exercise, and a balanced diet. She discovered that toxins—in cosmetics, clothing, cleaning products, auto exhaust, incinera-
tors, plastics, carpets, perfumes, and more—could affect her organs,
immune system, and every cell, including the brain. She had never
heard about toxins during the pink-ribbon cancer-awareness marches
and events. But her view changed as she started writing a book and
developing her organization (both called *Cancer Schmancer*) to trans-
form women from just cancer patients into knowledgeable medical
consumers. She would address all the areas where women could take
action to prevent illness, and avoiding toxins was at the top of the list.

Women and Toxins

Shouldn't concern about toxins be the same for boys and girls alike?
Apparently not. Women show more susceptibility to toxins for two
reasons. On one hand, women's bodies have more fat, where toxins
accumulate, so women are four times more likely to exhibit symptoms

of chemical sensitivity than men.[210] Women's lifestyles also put them in frequent contact with toxins, in the following ways:

Cosmetics. Chemical combos color our skin, eye-lashes, and lips; smooth wrinkles and plump contours; peel off the top layer from the skin; and remove oil, pollutants, and the makeup we applied.

Hair products. Gels, dyes, and sprays keep hair straightened, curled, extended, bleached, colored, conditioned, and in place, all while looking completely natural.

Nail products. Polish and acrylic fingernails are bonded to our nails and then removed by products that have longer warning instructions than directions for use.

Parenting. We drive our children on freeways, wait behind idling cars to pick them up after school, and sit for hours on playing fields treated with pesticides and herbicides.

Dry cleaning. We pick up dry cleaning and release the solvents in the closet of our bedrooms.

Shopping. We spend more time shopping,[211] exposing ourselves to more preservatives in new clothes[212] and toxins in new shoes.

Household cleaning products. The majority of us still clean our own houses, and we use cleaning products with potent chemicals—as do our housecleaners (who are usually women), if we're lucky enough to have them.

Jobs. We work in "pink collar" jobs, such as retail, nail care, and housecleaning, all of which expose us to the toxins described above, as well as office jobs, where we encounter printers and toners.

Let's face it. Toxins are unavoidable. They're in our food, water, air, playgrounds, and even in shampoo and makeup.

Toxins are a major contributing factor to the chronic death of your brain neurons. And since cells in the nervous system can't regenerate like other cells, we have to protect our neurons by avoiding exposure. Toxins can affect your mental abilities (memory, thinking, concentration, language, attention, and reaction time), physical problems (creating sleep issues, fatigue, headache, sexual dysfunction, developmental delays, and numb hands and feet), emotional issues (including depression, confusion, personality changes), behavior (contributing to irrational, criminal, or violent behavior), and illnesses (including movement disorders, multiple sclerosis, and chemical sensitivity).

Back in the 1700s, you'd have encountered natural toxins such as deadly nightshade plants, and toxic illnesses such as smallpox, tetanus, and polio. In the twenty-first century, we grapple instead with man-made chemicals and pollution. There are no vaccines to build immunity to these toxins, just experience and research to guide our choices.

However, data on the effects of toxins is not straightforward. Research on human subjects isn't easy. More often than not, people are exposed to multiple toxins at the same time, rather than one at a time. So it's difficult to isolate one toxin to understand its repercussions and safest dose. And do you know anyone who's never been exposed to any chemicals at all? I didn't think so. That means we can't conduct a definitive random controlled trial, comparing someone exposed to someone who hasn't been.

Instead, we have to learn from individuals who have various histories of health problems, medication use, and exposure to one or many chemicals simultaneously.

We're also learning in labs. But scientists in labs can't accurately mimic the complicated and amazing nature of the human nervous system. It can sometimes compensate for toxin exposure by creating new connections, but can also *decompensate* by breaking down neurons (neuro-degeneration) much later on.

Because we have a contaminated scientific playing field, data is easily manipulated and controversial. Chemical manufacturers, under the guise of for-health nonprofit organizations, can hire scientists to put a good spin on questionable products.

Becoming a Less Toxic Person

Even though you can't avoid toxins, you can make choices that can keep your brain, body, and family healthier.

It's true, some organic and truly natural products are more expensive. And the label "natural" or "green" may just be a figment of a marketing staff's imagination. But you can choose to use less of a more dangerous item, dilute it, mix it with a natural product (I do that with dishwasher soap), and/or change your standards of what is perfectly clean or perfectly attractive. You don't have to disdain makeup, but you might not aim for the look of Angelina Jolie on the red carpet—especially when you see a close-up of what's on her skin.

To start living a less toxic life, here's what you might want to pay attention to.

Food

These toxins particularly affect your brain and heart (which affects the health of your brain).

Watch how much and what kinds of fish you eat. Fish (or fish oil) provides omega-3 amino acids, your brain's superfood, but you'll find high levels of mercury in tuna, swordfish, and all kinds of shellfish. Too much mercury can harm your immune system, to trigger, among other things, lethargy, headaches, and digestive problems. To find good-for-you fish with fewer toxins, check out the Environmental Working Group's online fish list (see the resources section for the website address).

Stick with organic chicken. Traces of arsenic have been found in nonorganic chickens,[213] and studies have revealed the presence of salmonella, antibiotics, and microbial toxins in them, too. Also in our chicken meat are the estrogen hormones from the nonorganic feed.[214] We need only our own estrogen, not extra from chicken feed.

Buy organic produce, because pesticides present in nonorganic produce can lead to cancer, as well as nervous system and reproductive system damage. While organic produce still contains toxins that are naturally found in our environment, the levels and kind of toxins are much safer.

Switch to non–rBGH milk, because recombinant bovine growth hormone (rBGH) has been linked with diabetes and hypertension, both of which can affect the brain.[215] It's also been linked with breast and colon cancer. Soy, rice, coconut, and almond milk are good alternatives, especially when they're enriched with calcium.

Reduce sweets and choose natural sugar instead of artificial sweeteners. Sweeteners containing aspartame lead to cell damage, headaches, and dizziness. Other artificial sweeteners not containing aspartame claim to be completely safe, but your best bet is to just avoid them all, including those found in diet sodas. Some say fruit-juice sweeteners and Stevia (a European favorite, made from a plant leaf) are better than refined sugar. Agave nectar may not be as healthy as was once thought.

Reduce canned foods, because cans are commonly lined with bisphenol-A, a compound linked with diabetes and heart disease.

Avoid processed meats. Sausage, salami, hot dogs, and bacon contain sodium nitrate as well as other harmful ingredients called nitrosamines, which can lead to cancer, including brain tumors.[216] Be moderate with naturally processed meats as well, as they may not be much healthier.

Cut back on dairy and meat products. Although many contaminants, like polybrominated diphenyl ethers and polychlorinated biphenyl and dioxins, have been banned, they're still present in the soil of the fields in which animals feed. These toxins can cause serious damage to the nervous system—which is why they were banned.[217]

Tobacco

Nicotine is more addictive than heroin, and smoking affects the brain like heroin use does: both stimulate the release of opioids and dopamine, which play a role in soothing pain, increasing positive emotions, and creating a sense of reward.[218]

But it's not all fun and games. Beyond the health affects you've heard of—heart and circulatory diseases; lung diseases, such as emphysema and bronchitis; cancers of the blood, bladder, pancreas, lung, throat, and kidney; reduced heart and lung capacity; bone loss; aging and wrinkles; and shortened life span—smoking is also downright brutal to the brain.

- A compound in tobacco triggers the brain's white blood cells to attack healthy brain cells.[219]

- Smoking thins out an area of the cerebral cortex that plays an important role in reward-processes, impulse control, and decision-making.[220]

- Carbon monoxide in cigarette smoke binds to the hemoglobin molecules in your red blood cells, reducing the amount of oxygen available to the brain—part of what creates smoking's euphoric high.

- Nicotine withdrawal leads to mood changes, irritability, and anxiety.

- Contrary to popular thinking, smoking does not help you concentrate. Researchers at the University of Michigan found that smokers lose mental speed and accuracy and lower their IQ.[221]

- Heavy smoking in midlife increases your risk of developing Alzheimer's disease by over 150%.[222]

It takes support, structure, and courage to quit smoking. And it often takes more than one try to completely quit. But you don't have to make changes alone. Check out online programs such as Smoke-free.gov and American Lung Associations' teen program Not on Tobacco (NOT). Your employer or health care plan may also provide phone and other support programs.

If you're going it alone, consider writing down your reasons and your plan for quitting, including your quit date. Enlist a friend to support or quit with you. Put up a picture of a family member with the note, "I'm quitting for myself and for you." Move—it's hard to smoke while biking or walking. Find something else to do when you have the urge to smoke, like putting a drinking straw in your mouth.

You can do it. I did.

Cell Phones

Are cell phones safe for your brain? Absolutely, says the cell-phone industry. There is no definitive link between cell-phone use and cancer or brain tumors, it says. But organizations like the Environmental Working Group (EWG) are not convinced.

Recent studies find a significantly higher risk of brain and salivary-gland tumors among people who have used cell phones for ten years or longer.[223] And new data from the National Institutes of Health suggests that cell-phone radiation affects brain activity: When the user in the study was on the phone for more than fifty minutes, the brain activity increased by about 7% in the regions closest to the antenna. The same data shows that the human brain is sensitive to the electromagnetic waves coming off of a cell phone.[224]

To keep your brain safe, avoiding or limiting cell-phone use is a good idea. Though it's pretty hard to live without a cell phone these days, you can:

- Turn off the phone when you don't need it on.

- Send text messages instead of making calls.

- Purchase a phone with a low specific absorption rate (SAR). The SAR is a way of measuring the quantity of radiofrequency (RF) energy that is absorbed by the body.

- Use a headset to reduce RF energy to the brain. Some say to use only air-tube headsets, as wired headsets may act as antennas. Others, such as the American Cancer Society, recommend wired headsets. Bluetooth can reduce the SAR, but manufacturers are not required to note RF emissions from headsets.

- Use cell phones only for short calls. Let children use them only in emergencies.

- If you carry a cell phone on your body, keep the motor away and the key pad facing in.

- Wait for the call to connect before placing the phone next to the ear.

- Do not make a call when the signal strength is one bar or less, which means the phone must work harder to establish a connection.

Beauty Products

About *half* of the personal care products available to us have at least one chemical linked to either reproductive problems or cancer, says the Environmental Working Group (EWG).[225] Look up your brand of personal products at EWG's Skin Deep website. It tells the products' levels of toxicity, ingredient descriptions, and potential concerns for over 10,000 ingredients on more than 30,000 products. It also lists products to avoid. Here are a few things to watch out for.

In cosmetics: Watch for the preservative *parabens,* which has been linked to breast tumors in women and, to a lesser extent, affects the blood-brain barrier and contributes to neurotoxicity (killing or disrupting neurons). On labels, the chemical can be listed as *ethylparaben, propylparaben,* and *methylparaben.*

In nail polish: Look out for phthalates, a plastic softener and solvent. Health advocates say that this chemical is also associated with potential reproductive problems, IQ issues in children,[226] and possible nerve toxicity (when used in fragrances).[227] But you may not be able to tell if a product contains phthalates—companies aren't always required to list them on product labels.[228] (See the plastics section of this chapter for more on phthalates.)

In sunscreen: Oxybenzone, an active ingredient in many sunscreen products, has been linked to biological or cellular changes to the skin, which could lead to heart disease, as well as possibly being toxic to the brain, and nervous and organ systems. It is also toxic to wildlife and the environment.[229] Many sunscreens also contain the preservative parabens.

In hair products: You apply their hazardous toxins, often a combination of oxybenzone and fragrance, close to your brain. Many fragrance chemicals are related to neurotoxicity, allergies, and immunotoxicity.

In anti-aging cream: EWG says Aveeno Active Naturals Positively Ageless Firming Eye Cream is highly hazardous (in 2010) because it contains fragrance and DMDM hydantoin, which is related to immunotoxicity and allergies.

Fragrances—included in moisturizer, shampoo, hair color and bleach, conditioner, body wash, facial moisturizer, styling gel, facial cleanser, and anti-aging skin-care products—can contain neurotoxins and are among the top five allergens ever.[230] However, federal law doesn't require companies to list any of the potentially hundreds of chemicals in a single product's fragrance mixture or nail polish on product labels, says the EWG.[231]

Cleaning Supplies

Women handle and inhale more poisonous cleaning products than men. They're exposed to dishwashing rinse agents that release chlorine and quarternium 15 (a chemical that releases formaldehyde); bleaches in counter cleaners and mildew remover; and other items that have ammonia, ethers, phosphates, and ethoxylated nonyl phenols, which can do things like induce female characteristics in male fish.[232]

Check out natural cleaning products, which are widely available. But you may want to look for which products actually clean the best by checking out reviews and *Consumer Reports* before you experiment yourself.

New Clothes and Textiles

You know how crisp and bright your new shirt is? And how it feels so fresh? Sadly, these new clothes are treated with preservatives like formaldehyde.[233] Fabrics typically treated with formaldehyde-based resins include rayon, blended cotton, corduroy, wrinkle-resistant 100% cotton, and synthetic-blended polymer fabrics.[234] Be sure to wash the clothes before wearing them, and wash new bedding, towels, and pillows before using them. And wash your hands after shopping.

Plastics, Including Athletic Shoes

Stinky plastics are from *PVC (polyvinyl chloride),* also known as vinyl, made with chlorine, heavy metals, and other toxic plasticizers. Making and incinerating vinyl produces dioxin, a potent carcinogen.

Beware of out-gassing, which occurs when the volatile toxic chemicals in a plastic evaporate out of the material into the air. You can smell those chemicals when you open a new shower curtain or Barbie doll package. If a plastic stinks when you open the package, air it outside. Or better yet, use other types of plastic instead.

For more on how to avoid harmful plastics, check out Cancer Schmancer's plastic dos and don'ts on its website (see the resources section).

Phthalates are known as endocrine disruptors because they mimic the body's hormones and have, in laboratory animal tests, been shown to cause reproductive and neurological damage. (California banned the use of phthalates in toys and baby products as of 2009.) Phthalates are flexible plastics, but they're not just in shower curtains and rubber duckies. They're in things like car dashboards, steering wheels, and gearshifts and are what give cars that new-car smell. They make fragrances linger longer, help lotions spread, and help keep color in makeup. You'll find them in lipstick, hairspray, deodorants, aftershave lotions, nail polish, and nail-polish remover.

What can you do to avoid phthalates? Avoid things that have "fragrance" listed in their ingredients lists; that fragrance is a compound that possibly includes phthalates. Also use plastics with the recycling code 1, 2, or 5, rather than codes 3 and 7, which contain phthalates. Check the Pollution in People website and its page "Reading Labels to Avoid Phthalates" (see the resources section) for more details.

There's More?

Unfortunately, yes. You can find these toxins all over: pesticides, herbicides, heavy metals such as lead and mercury, car exhaust, Perc from dry-cleaning solvents, PCBs (polychlorinated biphenyls) in electronic equipment, mold in your house, flame retardants (PDBEs, or polybrominated diphenylethers, in children's pajamas, foam, and television and computer casings), ammonia, carbonless copy paper, printer toner, carbon monoxide, chlorine, formaldehyde, gasoline, glue and adhesives, nicotine, paint, paint remover, radiation, chemotherapy drugs, and wood preservatives.[235]

But don't give up hope. The best way to avoid toxins involves three steps: (1) Decide what you're going to do to be a less toxic lady with a less toxic home, (2) do it, then (3) relax. Too much stress is toxic too. However, you can manage your stress level. When you get panicked about all the possible dangers lurking in every possible nook and cranny, just stop, take a breath, and let your brain rebalance itself. The brain can handle life's threats much better when you're calm.

Chapter 10

Electronics on the Brain
One Second, I Just Need to See This Text . . .

Computers are useless. They can only give you answers.

Pablo Picasso, artist

A Sunday *Pearls Before Swine* comic reminds us what we're up against.

"I will finish my resume," says the Rat, who sits in front of a computer.

Ping!

"Hey, I have an email," says the Rat. "Could be important . . . . Wow, it has a YouTube link—gotta watch. Look, there are more shows I've never seen before. I'll check this one in Wikipedia. Wait, that's not the right show, but that girl looks interesting. I'll Google Image her. Cool photos, I'll post them on Facebook—Hey! A friend request. Who is this guy? I should Google him. He's too weird, I'll write about him on my blog. Who's reading my blog? I'll Google myself.

"No, no, no, it's time to do my resume . . . ."

Ping!

"Ooh, an email!"

Sound familiar? We have created a culture where technology is eating us up and eating the attention of our brains. If you're feeling overloaded by emails, text messages, websites, social media, computer programs, and other electronic stimulation, it's not because you have a lacking or aging brain.

Your brain was designed to efficiently process one thing, one cognitive operation at a time. It was also designed to get breaks and to have separations, leaving work at work and home at home like we did a generation ago.

Now, our brains are expected to be everywhere, all the time. A recent survey of workplaces found that employees were distracted about every three minutes. Most had about eight windows open on their computers at a time,[236] and they changed windows or checked email or other programs nearly thirty-seven times an hour.[237] A study at Microsoft discovered that employees took fifteen minutes or more to return to a challenging task when they strayed in order to answer emails or return instant messages. That's an estimated productivity loss of as high as $650 billion per year.

Ironically, four giant software companies who created this overload—Microsoft, IBM, Google, and Intel—have formed the Information Overload Research Group to try to develop solutions to the overload problem for work.

Many think that they are "supertaskers." But in reality, when you try to do two things at once—like juggle an Excel spreadsheet while checking out Facebook—you have dual-task interference and lose information.

We have a central bottleneck for information processing; it's located in a neural network within the frontal lobes of our brain. It severely limits our ability to multitask, according to Vanderbilt University neuroscientists.[238] The bottleneck occurs because brain regions have to choose which task to respond to first. Your teen will experience dual-task interference when she's listening and singing along to and selecting music while doing homework. On the other hand, surgeons who just listen to music while working in the operating room don't have a bottleneck, because there no choice is involved.[239]

Distractions: The Land of No Return

Can you ignore the sound alert from your email program signaling that you have a new message? Most can't. In fact, your brain changes with all the interruptions and with screen time. Screen-based media strengthens visual-spatial intelligence, which is great for air-traffic controllers and those keeping track of lots of simultaneous signals. But that skill is accompanied by weaknesses in higher-order cognitive processes, critical thinking, reflection, inductive reasoning, and mindfulness, says Patricia Greenfield who studies how media affects learning at UCLA.[240]

The life of a high-tech zombie is one of *continuous partial attention*. When you're online, you feel pulled by the lure of social networking—the people-information stream. The term *continuous partial attention* was coined by Linda Stone, a former Microsoft and Apple executive who focuses on implications of computer use. With continuous partial attention, you're in a heightened monitoring state, looking for a connection to the world of community and information.

Have you ever felt the vortex of procrastination diffusing your focus on tasks? If so, you're operating in persistent high alert, says Stone, which compromises your ability to reflect, make decisions, and think creatively.[241] You never get really settled in what you're doing, because you follow the persistent distractions.

Modern technology is also causing symptoms similar to those of attention-deficit disorder (ADD). Dr. Edward Hallowell calls the condition attention-deficit trait (ADT).[242]

"You've become so busy attending to so many inputs and outputs that you become increasingly distracted, irritable, impulsive, restless and, over the long term, underachieving," says Hallowell, a leading expert on ADD and the author of *Driven to Distraction*. "We've been able to overload manual labor. But never before have we so routinely been able to overload [the brain circuitry and] brain labor."[243]

Multitaskers have more fractured thinking and trouble shutting out irrelevant information, even when they are offline. Nicholas Carr, author of "Is Google Making Us Stupid?" says that constant multitasking creates shallower thinking, weakened concentration, reduced creativity, and heightened stress.[224] Women have been multitasking forever—taking care of kids, house, and family, all while doing professional work. But electronic multitasking requires narrow focus and short attention, and our eyes are mesmerized by shifting lights and visual intensity.

Your Brain on Television

Ever been glued to your TV and wondered why it's so difficult to look away? Here's why: Visual interruptions demand our attention and compel us to get our bearings, according to Ivan Pavlov (1849–1936). He's the famous Russian physiologist who studied conditioned responses well before TV. Television's rapid visual cuts, zooms, and pans trigger this *orienting response* much faster than real life ever could. Your eyes stay glued to the screen, even during stupid commercials or when someone is trying to have an intimate conversation with you, because you're constantly trying to reorient yourself to the changing visuals and content. That's also why we end up watching the tube a lot longer than originally intended.[245]

How to Untether From Technology

Can you get more attentive, more efficient, and less addicted to technology? It's definitely possible.

Take a Break from the Internet

We need help—some of us more than others. Between 5 and 10% of Internet users suffer web dependency, says Maressa Orzack, director of the Computer Addiction Study Center at Harvard University's McLean Hospital.[246]

Now we have some computer programs to stop the onslaught, to help people to focus instead of fighting the gnats of distraction. Some software, like Ulysses, Writespace, Scrivner, WriteRoom, and DarkRoom, hides everything but a minimalist word processor. Other programs such as LeechBlock, Isolator, Turn Off the Lights, MenuEclipse, Think, and SelfControl eliminate distracting toolbars or turn off specific Internet programs, such as Facebook, email programs, and other mind-fluff, for a specified period of time.[247]

Freedom software for both Mac and PC goes whole-hog. You set it to lock you out of the Internet from fifteen minutes to eight hours.

To get back on, you can wait until the timer runs out, or you can reboot your computer—a hassle that you can avoid by staying on-task. Writer/director Nora Ephron uses Freedom, and so do I.

Withdraw

Withdraw in two steps, says William Powers, author of *Hamlet's Black-Berry: A Practical Philosophy for Building a Good Life in the Digital Age:* (1) Know why you're withdrawing from your devices; perhaps to be more focused or because you're simply not as alive as you could be. (2) Create a habit, like disconnecting from technology every weekend. It's hard at first, but easier when you connect with yourself and those around you.

Just Stop

In the *New York Times* "First Steps to Digital Detox," Nicholas Carr says the only way to stop is to stop: turn off the BlackBerry and the iPhone, and check e-mail only two or three times a day. Cutting back may be challenging at first, as you reframe how you manage career communications and an initial sense of social isolation. "At the very least, you'll probably feel calmer, sharper and more in control of your thoughts," says Carr.[248]

One Task at a Time

Turn off extraneous devices (do you have several of them on at once?), says Gary Small, director of the Memory and Aging Research Center at UCLA. Just do one task and one gadget at a time.

Balance Your Tech Time

Small suggests you "make an effort to balance your tech time with regular off-line breaks." Every hour or so, go low-tech and turn off your gadgets. Write a letter, have a conversation, take a walk, stretch. These no-tech breaks will minimize stress, maintain focus, and improve your quality of life.

Use Distractions Purposefully

Distractions do take us away from the present, but that can be useful at times. One time, soon after my husband and I started living together in 1989, he stayed out with friends much later than expected. My worry went into overdrive, and I started to imagine the worst of the worst. What helped? A word game—could have been Boggle—on our Macintosh SE/30, with a black-and-white, nine-inch screen. During the game I was calm and cool while I figured out words from the jumble of letters. As soon as the game ended, the rush of worry returned until I pressed "play again." This zone-out was just as comforting, but less fattening than a bag of Oreos.

For most of us, technology is driving the bus, and we've lost the humanness of ourselves. Even if you don't turn the tide of your whole office, whole house, or whole life, you can touch base with yourself regularly. Remember that you are not defined by your email, Facebook comments, text messages, or clever ability with Bejeweled.

Instead of letting technology rule you, use it. Set up passwords, schedule break times, and leave messages on your screen that remind you that you're an even more amazing invention than the computer. Notice and care for yourself.

Chapter 11

The Brain and Community
Getting by With a Little Help From Your Friends

*I would never belong to a group that would accept
someone like me as a member.*

Groucho Marx, comedian

Living together is an art.

William Pickens, linguist, writer, educator

Who's your best friend? Does she (or he): make you laugh; remember that you don't like Thai food; listen to your love-life soap opera; know that it still bugs you that your brother-in-law was rude at your wedding; send you a dumb over-the-hill birthday card each year; know that when you say, "Why did I have kids?!" you really love them; and remind you that even though you have become a better person over the decades, you are *still* kind of bossy? When you love your best friend, not only does your heart feel bigger, but that feeling is making your brain bigger, too, by generating an expanded neural network. Connecting with others stretches various parts of your brain, engages your creativity, and connects you with the larger world. Your brain loves community.

Connecting With Friends Connects Your Neurons

Do you feel that you are on the same wavelength as your friend? You might actually be. A study at Princeton revealed a few interesting things about communication and the brain. Brain scans show that a speaker and listener don't use separate parts of the brain; instead, they use common neural subsystems, and they synchronize their respective neural activity.[249]

That study is in the hot field of social neuroscience, which explores how the brain is involved with our social interactions. This cutting-edge research, says Chris Frith of the Institute of Neurology at University College in London, "is undoubtedly going to be the dominant theme in 21st-century neuroscience."[250]

Social interactions require a lot of the brain's abilities, including those not activated by simply reading, listening, or talking. Daniel Goleman, author of *Social Intelligence,* says these abilities range from social awareness (assessing feelings of others) to social facility (awareness and ability of presenting oneself).[251]

While we've only just begun understanding social neuroscience, we know a few ways interacting with others engages your brain.

Watching and Feeling

Mirror neurons respond to actions that we observe in others, firing as they would if we were doing the action ourselves.[252] At the very least, mirror neurons explain the fervor of couch athletes who wear a copy of their favorite player's uniform and of drivers belting out "Single Ladies" with the radio.

Scientists think that mirror neurons, located in many areas of the brain, help us understand people's feelings, intentions, and emotions, creating empathy.[253] V. S. Ramachandran, one of the most renowned neuroscientists in behavioral neurology, predicted that "mirror neurons would do for psychology what DNA did for biology."[254] They make emotions contagious. Goleman says these automatic understandings and reactions to others are "neural Wi-Fi."

Getting and Expressing Nonverbal Messages

Words make up only about 20% of our messages, and the rest is nonverbal—body language, facial expressions, and gestures. When you're conversing with someone, you're engaging your motor and visual cortices. Both the speaker and listener do even more nonverbal communication if there's helping, learning, or walking involved in their exchange.

Working With Words

When someone explains her idea, a plot of a movie, or what she did over the weekend, the brain's Wernicke's area (located in the left temporal lobe) makes meaning out of those strange sounds we call words. When you translate your own thoughts into speech, your brain's Broca's area (located in the lower portion of the left frontal lobe) creates meaningful words, grammar, and syntax—a complicated process of verbal fluency.[255]

Thinking

Your thinking brain works hard when you're connecting. When you're listening, the first thing your brain does is to make sure the messages are congruent. Do you believe your co-worker's smile when her eyes are frowning?

Second, your brain compares the message you receive with your own way of seeing the world. Does the message match or challenge your view? Third, your brain decides whether to assimilate the information, change your framework, or perhaps defend your point-of-view in response. This constant process while you exchange ideas requires a high-level synthesis of new information and conceptual frameworks.

Feeling

Social interaction can evoke emotion, which signals the brain to pay attention and remember something. The neurons in the limbic system fire at a higher-than-usual frequency to determine if the emotion/situation is good or bad, painful or pleasurable, an opportunity or a threat.

Do Facebook Friends Expand Your Brain?

The *Time Magazine* headline said, "More Friends on Facebook Equals a Bigger Amygdala in Your Brain."[256] Which is absolutely, kinda true. Except for the part about Facebook. And except that they don't know if having more friends causes a bigger amygdala or vice versa.

The study at Massachusetts General Hospital *has* verified that people with more complex social relationships also have larger amygdalae. (An example of a complex relationship is one where your friend is also your boss; you have to decide when to talk about programming specs and when to talk about her last date.[257]) The amygdala deals with emotions, helps process memories, and gets totally absorbed in managing our response to fear and stress. It may play a central role in coordinating our ability to size people up, remember names and faces, and handle a range of social acquaintances.

Those with the smallest amygdalae had fewer than five to fifteen people as regular contacts, while those with the largest listed up to fifty acquaintances in their social lives. A related study at Oxford theorized the maximum number of meaningful relationships the brain can handle is 150.[258] This limit could be why we have a hard time remembering names, since our brains are full of the names of celebrities, cars, and book authors. Older participants in the study tended to have smaller amygdalae and fewer people in their social group, perhaps because of death of friends, isolation due to illness, or withdrawal.[259]

Social Stimulation Lengthens Your Life

Social relationships predict a person's odds of living or dying. A Brigham Young University study says that increased social connections—having more friends, family, neighbors, or colleagues—improve our odds of survival by 50%. On the other hand, low social interaction carries the same health risk as smoking fifteen cigarettes a day or being an alcoholic; it is also as risky as not exercising and twice as risky as obesity.[260]

On the other hand, a separate study from Kaiser Permanente Health Care found that elderly women who maintained large social networks showed significantly less risk of dementia, and they delayed or prevented the onset of cognitive impairment.[261] However, the question still is whether having bigger social networks reduces dementia or having a reduced tendency for dementia allows for bigger social networks.

Even though we can't conclusively say that having friends reduces dementia, it's clear that it will stimulate your brain—even if you're just chatting with the cashier or postman—and hopefully make your life more enjoyable.

Create a Reservoir of Brain Function

If you build a stash of cognitive brain function, you can draw from it if other areas of your brain decline. A strong social fabric gives your brain a good workout and creates that cognitive stash to help protect your neurons.[262]

> *Socializing gives your brain a good workout and builds a stash of cognitive brain function.*

Surprisingly, even if social interactions don't change *the brains* of those with Alzheimer's, it can still change *brain functioning.* A study at Rush University Alzheimer's Disease Center evaluated eighty-nine elderly people with Alzheimer's on their level of everyday functioning and involvement with children, spouses, friends, and groups or organizations. The more socializing they did, the higher their brain functioning was.[263]

The really interesting result came up when researchers autopsied the subjects' brains after they'd died: *All* the brains were riddled with diseased plaques and tangles from the disease. But those with an active social life had some kind of protective reserve, so they could function better as the disease progressed.

Part of the benefit of socializing, theorizes Dr. Denise Park, director of the University of Texas Center for Vital Longevity, is that, like mental exercises and learning, it limits the amount of time that aging brains remain unfocused, in a daydream state. Socializing also strengthens the ability to switch between the daydream state and focused attention, enabling you to maintain a more productive and independent life.[264]

Socializing also strengthens your ability to switch between a daydream state and focused attention.

The Alzheimer's Association's Dr. William Theis says that science will reveal more and more how social interaction stimulates new connections in the brain. In the meantime, he recommends you do your usual healthy activities for the brain—learning new skills, going for a daily walk, or taking a dance class—in the company of friends.[265]

How to Expand Your People Network and Neural Network

There are many ways to increase your social connections and help your brain.

Be Engaged

No matter what you do, focus on being engaged with the people you're doing it with. Active listening—paraphrasing what someone says to make sure you understand it—activates your brain's executive function.

Plan to Connect

Create a routine with a group or a friend so you have fewer barriers to deciding whether or not to meet. Have a weekly or monthly walk, coffee, lunch, book reading, or just a date to browse what's new at the discount store.

For instance, I'm still part of a "new" parents group that's nineteen years old. We've continued because we have regular gatherings (no finagling with plans), with scheduled hosting duties according to the alphabetical order of our children's names, and the host cooks dinner for all the families (four free dinners in exchange for making just one huge meal every couple of months). We've created a supportive community, and—best friends or not—the brain and heart thrive on continuing social stimulation and connection.

Volunteer

Did you know that volunteering releases the "happy" neurotransmitter dopamine? Those who give are healthier, emotionally and even physically, than those who don't, because volunteering increases your sense of well-being and reduces stress.[266] Add to that the stimulation to your brain, and you have all the motivation you need to sign up.

If you haven't come up with good volunteer opportunities, check your region's United Way branch to match your skills, schedule, and location with options. (Their opportunities to volunteer are usually on the Internet.) Aim to find an opportunity where you are working with others and perhaps learning a new skill.

Play Games With Others

There's a reason that chess, checkers, mah-jongg, and even bingo have been popular for years. They're fun, and they stretch the social and cognitive brain. Form or find a group that plays pinochle, poker, or Pictionary at homes or coffee shops. Check postings at bookstores and coffee houses.

Join a Group

Want to talk, learn, or get support for writing, an illness, politics, addictions, music, fandom, business referrals, transitions, atheism, adoption, cooking, or just about anything else? Join a club on a topic that can stretch your thoughts. Book clubs are a great place to start (check your library). Or try a civic or politics club (especially ones that debate different sides), environmental group, religious or spiritual group, Toastmasters, or even a lecture where you can pipe in a question. The "group" section of Craigslist is worth a look, though you may want to meet in a public place until you get to know the folks first.

Move

You'll hit the jackpot for the brain when you combine social and physical activity: row crew with others, join a class or gym that encourages introductions, join a training-support group at a nonprofit with an upcoming marathon or event, join a club for swimming or other sport, take up dancing, become a dragon boater, volunteer at a community garden, or walk and talk with a friend.

Use Technology Well

On the one hand, Goleman says, technology has made it easier to disconnect from those around us, as well as from ourselves, if we rely on it instead of face-to-face discussions for communication. With just short bits of conversations, the brain doesn't stretch to integrate information, come up with responses, or monitor feedback from facial expressions or tone of voice. Technology could be making us socially stupider.

On the other hand, you can use technology—headsets on phones, specifically—to connect with friends while you're folding clothes, making lunch, or cleaning the clutter from the coffee table. That's the way women used to connect long ago, by doing chores together, and now we can do it while on the phone. It's not the same as talking while you're relaxed on the couch, but it's better than never talking at all because you're too busy.

When you are online, make stronger connections: show your passion, be a connector, give thanks and help, and join chats or webinars where people talk about a topic for a longer time.

Address Shyness

If you're shy, you can still find ways to connect or use your social brain. Volunteer or join classes; then you can chat about the task at hand, instead of navigating small talk. If you like animals, volunteer at an animal shelter, or take your pet to a dog park, where it's easy to converse about the mud or how fast a dog runs. Even talking aloud to your dog stimulates your brain.

Make New Friends and Keep the Old

Navigating friendships may include some losses with the gains. For instance, a friend you were close with for years suddenly has no time because of family or work obligations, or sadly has a change of heart about your connection. Grieve the loss and make new connections. New friends may not know where you went to elementary school, but they can enhance your life in other ways.

Sure, making social connections, opening up your brain and heart, is a risk. After all, you could experience a loss. But when you connect, you learn about the world and about yourself in ways you can't get from reading, electronic social networks, or spending time alone.

Be generous with yourself and your connections. Your brain will be happier, but beyond that, you will have some company on your journey on this planet. That's not a small thing: even when people leave, the connection never really goes away.

Find somebody to love, like, dislike, or just talk with—share yourself. Both you and your brain will get back more than you imagine.

Chapter 12

Aging, Alzheimer's, and the Brain
Did I Read This Already?

One keeps on forgetting old age up to the very brink of the grave.

Colette, novelist

Age is a question of mind over matter.
If you don't mind, it doesn't matter.

Satchel Paige, baseball player

You and your lovely brain are getting older.

On the one hand, your brain is getting better, making more connections, and savoring its plasticity. If you age without any sort of neuron or brain disease, most if not all of your neurons will remain healthy until you die.

On the other hand, your brain gets pretty messy when it ages, even without disease. The brain shrinks, losing 5 to 10% of its weight between ages twenty and ninety. The decaying parts of your dendrites (those treelike branches that extend from neurons to stimulate connections) get more tangled, so it's harder to make connections. Any damaged or dying neurons form hard chunks of senile plaques, and there's no brain hygienist to clean them off.

Genetics are a key factor in determining how you age, but you're not just at the mercy of your parents. You can slow down brain aging in a few ways, like keeping a lower body weight. One reason maintaining a healthy weight helps might be that it lowers blood-glucose levels. "Blood glucose is a very reactive chemical and can cause damage to proteins," including proteins that get your brain up and running says Caleb Finch, PhD, who studies the neurobiology of aging at the University of Southern California.[267]

You can also keep your brain healthier as you age by:

Moving more. Regular physical activity prevents age-related brain fogginess, says Dr. John Ratey, author of *Spark*.

Doing mentally engaging activities. Play games. Push beyond safe limits to stretch your neurons into making more connections. On the computer, try matching, word, or brain games.

Drinking water and **eating colorful veggies and fruits.**

Eating chocolate. Oxford University discovered that people who enjoy chocolate in moderation scored higher on memory tests than those who didn't indulge.[268]

Drinking a little beer or wine. One beer each day can help reduce the risk of mini strokes, and a glass of wine or spirits can reduce risk of dementia.[269] But if you go too far, you can damage your brain with alcohol and increase your risk.

Chilling out. Counter stress with relaxation and calm words.

Staying connected and socializing. Social stimulation and conversations stretch your brain connections. So does laughter.

Alzheimer's: When the Brain Loses Hold

No one wants to suffer pain or illness, but losing mental capacity is near the top of most people's lists of things they'd like to avoid as they age. And many fear their brains will lose hold because of Alzheimer's disease.

It's hard to avoid hearing about Alzheimer's: 30% of Americans have a family member with the disease, and most of the caregivers (60%) are women. In 2010, over 5,000 news stories were released on Alzheimer's and its research.

The research is interesting—and confusing. For instance, 65% of those with Alzheimer's are women, according to the 2010 Alzheimer's Association study. Turns out, the frequency of Alzheimer's in women is not greater than it is in men.[270] The statistics appear higher because "women live in a longer period in an age of risk," said Dr. Soo Borson, director of the Memory Disorders Clinic at the University of Washington and presenter on the PBS series *The Art of Aging*. Women live longer than men, comprising 58% of people over age sixty-five, and 67% of those over eighty-five in the U.S.[271] "Age, not gender is the preponderant cause of Alzheimer's, said Borson. "Women don't have a higher incidence at any given age point."

Before we get into more Alzheimer's research and statistics, let's define what it is and what it does to the brain.

How Alzheimer's Affects the Brain

Alzheimer's destroys neurons and other brain cells, disrupts the way electrical charges travel within cells, and disrupts the activity of neurotransmitters.[272] Plaques, abnormal clusters of protein, build up between nerve cells. Shrinking, dead, and dying nerve cells contain tangles, which are made up of twisted strands of another protein. The brain shrinks, and the shrinkage affects nearly all its functions, including thinking, planning, and remembering.

Alzheimer's usually lasts eight to ten years, and in most people with Alzheimer's, symptoms first appear after age sixty, says the Alzheimer's Association.[273] The stages of the disease are impairment, severe dementia, and failure to thrive.

Some doctors can diagnose Alzheimer's with a spinal tap or MRI, (though generally it takes a biopsy to be sure) but many don't want to, because they don't patients to worry about having a disease that has no cure. Doctors can also make sure memory problems are not from other problems: illnesses, head injuries, brain tumors, stroke, Parkinson's, hypothyroidism, hypoglycemia, nutrition or vitamin deficiencies, dehydration, kidney or liver failure, medication side effects, alcohol use, depression, trauma, or infections.

These symptoms, from the Alzheimer's Association, can help you sort out your normal brain farts from the disease's symptoms:[274]

Normal Life Problems That Happen Occasionally	Alzheimer's Symptoms
Forgetting a name or appointment, but remembering later	Memory loss that disrupts daily life
Errors when doubling a recipe or balancing a checkbook	Planning or problem-solving challenges
Needing help setting the microwave or working the TV remote	Difficulty completing familiar tasks at home or work
Temporary disorientation about the day of the week	Confusion with time or place
Vision changes related to new glasses or cataracts	Trouble understanding visual images and spatial relationships
Trouble finding the right word	New problems with words when speaking or writing (such as calling a watch a hand-clock")
Misplacing things from time to time	Misplacing things and losing the ability to retrace steps
Making a bad decision	Decreased or poor judgment
Feeling burnt out from work, family, and social obligations	Withdrawal from work or social activities
Getting irritated when your way of doing things gets disrupted	Changes in mood and personality

Brain Fitness for Women

Scientists are not absolutely sure what causes cell death and tissue loss in the Alzheimer brain, but those plaques and tangles are prime suspects. They may be connected with the inflammatory processes associated with aging, according to recent research.

Researchers are on a quest to understand what affects Alzheimer's and its progression, especially since between 2010 and 2030, 10,000 baby boomers will turn sixty-five each day. But some of these studies open themselves to questions as well.

Alzheimer's Research: Does It Keep Your Brain Together?

Could you avoid Alzheimer's if you took fish-oil supplements . . . ate healthy foods . . . got adequate vitamins (especially vitamin E and folic acid) . . . drank juice . . . ate curries . . . did Sudoku and crossword puzzles . . . read something challenging daily . . . engaged in a debate . . . turned off the TV . . . surfed the Internet . . . wrote in a daily journal . . . played Nintendo and brain-fitness games . . . changed it up and did something different . . . controlled cholesterol and high blood pressure . . . got enough sleep . . . didn't do drugs . . . cut alcohol consumption . . . took "statins" or selective estrogen receptor molecules . . . didn't smoke . . . meditated . . . thought positive thoughts . . . reduced stress . . . did neurofeedback . . . listened to music . . . hung out with friends . . . supported your marriage . . . avoided vaccines and other potential sources of mercury . . . avoided aluminum . . . and put vinegar in everything? All these things might make you healthier, but do any of them prevent Alzheimer's?

Many studies showing associations between activities and Alzheimer's often are "not stated with validity," says Borson. This was confirmed by a National Institutes of Health's State-of-the-Science conference in April 2010, which reviewed the results of both randomized control trials (the best of all study types) and observational studies on humans done over the last years.

The studies didn't find good evidence that supported what you can do to definitely modify the risk of Alzheimer's. Why? Some studies focused on a totally separate outcome, such as cancer or cardiovascular disease; some didn't have consistent ways to measure for Alzheimer's; or some measured the level of cognitive decline only once, which doesn't give a clear picture since the level doesn't decline step-by-step.

Actually, Alzheimer's is hard to measure because the brain, even in decline, is very smart. Its *cognitive reserve* makes it resilient and able to counteract damage. This reserve can be very useful to individuals, but it can hide evidence of pathological changes in studies.

With all that, what do we know about what affects Alzheimer's?[275] Let's start with the factors that are consistently associated with *increased* risk:

> **Smoking,** but there is no consistent evidence on past smoking,
>
> **High blood pressure, metabolic syndrome** (a cluster of medical abnormalities), and **diabetes,**
>
> **A gene variation** (ApoE) linked with increased types of cognitive decline.

These factors are associated with *reduced* risk for Alzheimer's and/or cognitive decline:

> **Light to moderate alcohol intake,**
>
> **Leisure activities,** such as painting, gardening, religious and club membership,
>
> **Cognitive training** (a five- to six-week training period), even to a modest extent five years after the training ends,
>
> **Diets low in saturated fat, Mediterranean diets,** and **high vegetable intake,**
>
> **Omega-3 fatty acids (fish oil),**
>
> **Increased physical activity,** including walking,
>
> **Learning a second language.** Bilingual people with Alzheimer's were diagnosed four years later than those who were monolingual. Even when their brains were not as healthy as those of monolingual people with the disease, the bilingual people functioned better.[276]

There is a link between depression and Alzheimer's, but "it is unclear whether . . . depression might reflect early features [symptoms] of Alzheimer's disease," says the study report. Meditation was not researched at the NIH State-of-the-Science conference, but studies have shown that it helps strengthen neural connections, thereby enhancing memory and improving focus. However, these studies were not related to Alzheimer's.

Many things have been said to help or be associated with Alzheimer's, but so far there isn't enough scientific evidence to back up the claims of the following items:

- Vitamin B-12, E, and C; folic acid; flavanoids; multivitamins; beta-carotene and ginkgo biloba;
- Obesity, sleep apnea, and traumatic brain injury;
- Socioeconomic status or years of education;
- Statins; antihypertensive or anti-inflammatory medications; cholinesterase inhibitors;
- Hormone replacement therapy (evidence is contradictory);
- Herbal preparations, toxins, or environmental exposures.

The next step will hopefully be more high-quality studies specifically for Alzheimer's, and many are in the works. For example, an interesting twelve-year study from Rush University Medical Center in Chicago has showed that brain exercise slowed mental decline, but then sped up dementia later in old age, reducing the overall amount of time that a person may suffer.[277]

When it comes to the brain and Alzheimer's, there is always more to learn. Borson, who has worked with brains for forty years says, "We have to have respect for the brain, nature, and its secrets. We really haven't cracked most of them."

Life With No Guarantees

How do you handle concerns about aging, Alzheimer's, and losing your cognitive power when there are no guarantees?

Live life as fully as possible. That means doing all the things that keep you engaged and healthy—move more, eat well, socialize, don't smoke, worry less, and keep yourself and your brain active. At the very least, that helps you maintain a healthy weight and prevent disease— and you may also reduce your risk of Alzheimer's and other age-related brain changes. At the very best, you will make this life, right now, a better one.

Chapter 13

Beyond the Mind

Expanding Your Connection
With Nature and Spirit

Let your mind be as a floating cloud. Let your stillness
be as a wooded glen. And sit up straight. You'll never meet
the Buddha with such rounded shoulders.

Sayings of the Jewish Buddhist

For one week each year, Stephanie remembered she was more than her brain. That was the second week of her vacation by the sea.

The first week, she cooked gourmet meals, drove her kids to miniature golf, and cleaned sand tracked into the rug. The second week, though, the "good vacation" no longer mattered. Instead of focusing on details, she had a sense of bigness surrounding everything. The stuff of vacation wasn't as important as being—with each other, with the ocean, with herself, with just the forces of life.

Stephanie didn't realize that "bigness" was good for her brain. And she could create it even during regular daily life.

Experiencing a connection with something bigger changes how the brain reacts. Regardless what you call the bigger force—nature, God, All That Is, Mohammed, Essence, Jesus, Krishna—the connection with it strengthens the prefrontal cortex. This front-most part of your brain is in charge of executive functions, like making moral choices, predicting your future events, and executing social control. Think of it as the grown-up part of your brain.

The brain also has a latent function that's triggered when you go beyond the mind—beyond how you subjectively perceive the world. Your limbic system tells the rest of your brain, "Let's experience the supernatural." Then your brain moves into hyperarousal, and you lose your sense of "I." Thoughts of yourself dissipate and are replaced by the experience of objective or bigger reality.

How do you go beyond the ordinary perceptions of the mind? Meditation, prayer, and experiencing nature can open doors.

Meditation Is Easy (Unless It's Not)

Okay, show of hands. How many have tried meditation? About 70% of Americans, according to *Time Magazine*.[278] And how many have stopped? I'm guessing nearly that many. People try meditation after hearing how great it is. Then they stop—likely because they get bored, forget, don't have time, or feel they're doing it wrong.

A new perspective on meditation can help you try it again or for the first time. And given how meditation benefits your brain and daily life, trying again is well worth it.

How Meditation Helps the Brain

Science began examining the experience of meditation in the 1970s. New technology in the last two decades has provided deeper information on brain waves and blood flow, helping research uncover what parts function in a meditating brain, the waves it produces, and how the body and cognition respond.

In 2003, Richard Davidson, a professor at the University of Wisconsin, and several others measured meditation's effects on mental and physical health, using a randomized controlled study. After research subjects did just eight weeks of regular meditation, they experienced highly beneficial effects—not only in their brains, but also in their immune function.

In 2005, the Dalai Lama held a gathering of neurologists and monks to publicly discuss the neuroscience of meditation. Sitting on the panel was Davidson. The neurologists solidified the Dalai Lama's claim that meditation can help us understand and alleviate certain kinds of human suffering, as the foundation for inner peace.

Dr. Andrew Newberg, a neuroscientist at the University of Pennsylvania, studied the effects of prayer on the brain. "The more you focus on something," he says, "whether that's math or auto racing or football or God—the more it becomes written into the neural connections of your brain." In one Tibetan Buddhist's brain, Newberg saw how the frontal lobes lit up on the brain scanner while the parietal lobes went completely dark. The parietal lobes allow us to understand our sense of self. Turning them off in meditation and prayer seems to allow us to make fewer separations to feel oneness with the universe.

Collectively, researchers agree that meditation has a measurably beneficial impact on the brain. If you practice it regularly, you can actually train your brain to enhance awareness, neural coordination, memory, and mental focus.

People who meditate regularly have *more* neural fibers in the frontal lobe. This area of the brain creates the qualities that make us beautiful human beings: integrity, compassion, unconditional love, sympathetic joy, awareness, and presence.

If meditation were a gadget on a TV infomercial, it'd be sold out right away. Fortunately, you don't have to give your credit card number to get these additional benefits associated with regular meditation:

- Physical and mental relaxation;
- An awareness of how feelings and thoughts come and go;
- Increased mental focus (mindfulness) and concentration;
- Improved attention;[279]
- Help recovering from psychosis;[280]
- Sensory experience;
- An awareness of how you narrate your life instead of noticing it (for example, telling yourself, "I need to describe this gorgeous sunset back at work");
- An awareness of something other than your thoughts;

- A greater connection with the world around you;
- A sense of detachment (for example, calmly watching yourself when you get frustrated, worried, bored, or overwhelmed instead of drowning in the feeling itself);
- Reduced stress;
- A stronger immune system;[281]
- Improved heart and digestive health;
- More calm and less anxiety, anger, and/or depression;[282]
- Improved frontal-lobe functioning, including problem solving, memory, language, and, judgment;[283]
- Increased compassion and loving kindness, happiness and peace;
- Sanity.

All this with just one twenty-minute session of counting your breath? Yes and no. You'll feel more relaxed with just one session—even more productive, efficient, and calm. But to get the most out of meditation means a regular practice.

Doing Meditation

Common meditation techniques include watching the breath, chanting a mantra, saying *om*, walking, concentrating on an image, and being aware of your senses and the moment. In meditation you are actually practicing doing nothing but one thing at a time.

What makes meditation hard is your mind—your wonderful, active, curious, intelligent, worried, daydreaming, productive mind. From your mind's perspective, it knows what's best. It can actually be a bit of a bully. And sitting and doing nothing? Not the best, says the mind.

The mind is a marvelous thing, but when it's in charge, it's like someone's directing a movie of your life. If there's a creak on the stairs when you're home alone at night, your mind shows you a private screening of the movie *Psycho* by Alfred Hitchcock. Your mind convinces you that waiting in line at the bank is as boring as watching a PowerPoint presentation describing human-resource regulations. Or your mind sees a wedding with the man you just met instead of the wedding ring on his finger.

Meditation on the other hand, gives you the gift of awareness, the realization that your mind, with its thoughts and story of your life, is not giving you the whole picture.

That gives you options. Instead of the *Psycho* movie, you can separate the sounds around you from those inside your head. While waiting in line, you can notice your breath and body. Instead of instant weddings, you can notice love is everywhere, not just in one person.

Meditation gets your mind out of the driver's seat and into the passenger seat. Then what drives? People say a variety of things: awareness, consciousness, the bigger picture, God, or a mystery. You get to find out for yourself.

How to Meditate

In reality it's not easy to do one thing without your mind wanting to do something else, says Ragini Michaels, author of *Unflappable: 6 Steps to Staying Happy, Centered, and Peaceful No Matter What*. Training your mind to focus is a big part of meditation. You also get to see what your mind really does: cling, want, judge, deny, avoid, distract, and try to control life.

How do you tame this "monkey mind," as many Buddhist traditions refer to it? With consistency. Sit down, close your eyes, and focus on counting your exhalations. When you find yourself thinking about going to the bank, buying coffee at the store, and worrying if you can pay your student loans, notice that your mind has wandered. Bring it back to your exhalations, and start with the count of one again.

Focus.

The mind wanders.

Notice that it has.

Bring your focus back to your meditation.

Even if you notice only at the end of a meditation that your mind wandered the entire time, you're doing meditation right. You're noticing. Every time you pull your mind back to your focus, you become more aware of how the mind drives your life, catching you in concepts or stories. When you notice, you return to experiencing life right here in this very moment.

---

*Even if you only notice at the end of a meditation
that your mind wandered for the entire time,
you're doing meditation right.*

You can start "doing nothing" right now. Can you hear rain on the roof, see colors of tulips, taste the soup you're eating, or feel your breath? Decide what you're going to focus on and, like Nike says, *just do it*. But remember, don't expect to do it perfectly. Just keep coming back to your focus.

Types of Meditation

All types of meditation involve focusing your mind; the difference is what each asks you to focus on. Your object of focus can include:

The breath. It's always there, moving in and out of your body. Experiencing your breath takes you into your body and connects you to the air outside of you. To stay focused, you can repeat, "Inhale, exhale" with each breath. Or count each exhale (or inhale), and return back to one after you reach ten—or anytime you get distracted. Become aware of the full breath in your body, feeling it at tip of your nose, filling your abdomen and chest, expanding your ribs and collarbone, and then releasing. You may want to focus on one area that's moved by your breath.

The pauses in your breath. Notice the empty moment at the end of the exhale, right before you breathe in again. And notice the pause at the end of the inhale, before the out-breath. You may find a moment of no thought and perhaps the experience of emptiness and expansion.

Compassionate thoughts. Repeat thoughts of compassion. Focus on yourself, people you love, people you like, people you don't know, and/or people you have animosity toward. Say or think, "May you (or I) be happy. May you be healthy. May you be safe. May you be free from suffering." These are phrases from *metta,* or loving-kindness meditation. Some find it challenging to extend those wishes to people they dislike—or to themselves. But compassionate meditation increases your connection and empathy for others.

A phrase. In transcendental meditation and other forms of meditation, you repeat a phrase or *mantra* in your head. The phrase can be passed down from a spiritual tradition, or it can be something familiar, such as, "My will is Thy will," "Shalom," or "Peace."

A prayer. The rosary, a Sufi Zikr, the Jewish *Shema, Om Mani Padme Hun,* or even a song like "Tis a Gift to Be Simple" can be points of focus.

A chant. Chanting is repeating a particular sound, such as *om,* or prayer aloud.

An object. Focus on a physical object—such as a piece of quartz, cross, or yoga symbol—and imagine or sense its essential nature, say Joel and Michelle Levy, authors of *Luminous Mind.* You can also picture the object or any other image in your mind's eye, focusing your attention to sharpen your mind.

Walking. As you walk, pay attention to each aspect of each footstep, from the change of balance, the initial release of the foot, its movement in space, gravity in the standing foot, your foot's placement on the ground. As you might expect, a walking meditation is a slow walk. In a faster walk, pay attention to one foot or one action in your movement (such as your changing balance).

Movement. Repetitive movements in qi gong, tai chi, and Osho moving meditations allow you to focus your awareness. Repeated movements in yoga, such as a series of sun salutations, can lead to a more meditative focus.

Sensations. Be aware of one sensation—sounds and silences, the breeze on your skin, the pressure of your behind on the chair, or the feel of feet in your shoes.

Or use soft focus as you look down at a point in front of you or concentrate on, say, the waves of the ocean. Contemplate the taste and texture of food transforming in your mouth.

Other points of focus. During any of your everyday activities, stay with one focus. If you swim for exercise, focus on your arm leaving and entering the water. Write ever so slowly as you fill in a crossword puzzle, focusing on the sensation of the pen creating each part of each letter. Notice the sensations of being with your partner or child, without planning, reminiscing, or fixing. Let your thoughts, interpretation, and narration of life be in the background of your awareness.[284]

Whichever object of focus you choose, use the same one over several weeks or months as you practice meditating. That deepens the practice.

How Often to Practice

Do you have to meditate for twenty minutes a day or twice a day? If you do, your brain will be thrilled. But just as your meditation doesn't need to be perfect, neither does the amount of time or the way you do it. You can meditate on the bus or in your car before work. Or you can just pause for a moment—maybe waiting in line at the grocery store—and notice life outside your thoughts: the colors and shapes of the signs, the smells, the sound of the cash register beeping. Any type of focus, done for any amount of time, leads you out of your mind and connects you to a bigger picture.

Any type of meditative focus leads you out of your mind and connects you to a bigger picture, no matter how long you do it.

On the other hand, the more you practice meditation, the more you'll train your brain to focus—and the less your awareness and focus will be swept away by thoughts of past events, future plans, or analysis-paralysis. In everyday life, it helps you be more able to stay with the sales report at work even as your cube neighbor talks on about last night's football game. Meditation doesn't make thoughts disappear. It provides another view so you can choose whether or not to pay attention to each one—and that expands your brain.

Prayer and the Brain

Prayer is closely related to meditation in many ways, says Patricia Carrington, PhD, author of *The Book of Meditation*. Both are contemplative and often done in quiet or solitude. In prayer, as in certain kinds of meditation, words and phrases—the rosary, the name of God—may be chanted. The body may have a special posture, and eyes are often closed.[285] "Used as a form of silent inner communion, or coupled with a mantra-like repetition of religious words," says Carrington, "prayer can be seen to blend imperceptibly into meditation." And like meditation, prayer can increase your connection with something bigger.

However, prayer may commonly be a "goal-directed activity," continues Carrington. "A person calls upon a deity to give praise or offer thanks; seek forgiveness, consolation or assistance; or enter into some other relationship." Meditation, she says, is "non-striving and relatively goal-less."

Neuroscientists have conducted studies about the brain and repetitive prayer. Andrew Newberg, author of *How God Changes Your Brain,* studied brain activity of praying Franciscan nuns, Pentecostals speaking in tongues, and Sikhs chanting. He found that these prayers increased whole-brain communication and lessened blood flow to the parietal lobes.[286]

"Improvised" or nonritual prayers of Danish Christians also activated a strong response in the brain in fMRIs (functional magnetic resonance imaging) studies. Activity increased in social cognition areas of the brain—the temporopolar regions, prefrontal cortex, and more—as shown by their blood-oxygen-level dependence.[287]

What do these changes in brain activity mean? As mentioned earlier, the parietal lobe creates a sense of self in the world, of time and space—"I have to shop first, drive to pick up the kids, and then cook dinner." As prayer reduces blood flow to these brain areas, you focus less on making your way in the world. Instead, Newberg says, you form more new connections, blurring boundaries between the self and other—"I stop and feel my breath and notice that my husband, the cat, trees, every living thing is doing some kind of breathing."[288]

Just like meditation, prayer renews your brain, meaning you increase your creativity, memory, and focus—all while you're reducing stress.

Prayer renews your brain, increasing your creativity, memory, and focus while reducing stress.

Newberg says that just thinking about God is great for the brain. "If you contemplate something as complex or mysterious as God," he says, "you're going to have incredible bursts of neural activity firing in different parts of your brain." He adds that new dendrites (those treelike parts of nerve cells that conduct nerve impulses) rapidly grow and old associations disconnect as you gain new imaginative perspectives.

People in prayer, from Sikhs to Pentacostals, experienced similar spiritual connections—no matter how they defined God or their religion.

"In essence," Newberg says, "when you think about the really big questions in life—be they religious, scientific, or psychological—your brain is going to grow."

Biophilia and the Brain

The Pacific Northwest has the lowest percentage of churchgoers in the United States. The common excuse people give for not going to church is, "I'd rather go for a hike in the mountains."

Are they just lazy? Not from the perspective of *biophilia,* the theory that the human brain is in love *(philia)* with nature *(bio).* While the name was coined in 1984 by renaissance biologist E. O. Wilson, research on how nature affects the brain is just beginning. I couldn't find any studies on how being in nature affects brain waves, but I did find plenty of studies that showed how natural scenes and architecture affect thinking, stress, healing, and memory. The nonprofit Príhatín Institute, on its website, cites studies supporting the following:

- Office workers have less stress if they have window views of natural landscapes.[289]

- Watching a tank of tropical fish reduces blood pressure and increases relaxation (which explains why so many dentists have them).[290]

- Post-surgery patients who could see a natural scene from their windows recovered more quickly than those without views of nature.[291]

- Cognitive processing improves by a brief walk outdoors, viewing nature through a window, and even being around indoor plants.[292]

Long-distance views, according to NASA research, calm down the mind, creating "cognitive tranquility."[293] Images of landscapes in photographs and posters have a calming effect and help people maintain their mental performance in high-stress environments. Even silk plants promote positive moods and reduce stress, says researcher Roger Ulrich.[294]

From taking a trip to the Grand Canyon to pulling a common weed, there are many ways to connect with nature.

> **On a daily basis,** you can put plants, pictures of landscapes, or an aquarium in your home or office; walk to a park on a break; notice the changes of the day, from the sunset to the stars at night to the morning dew; cuddle a pet; and love and appreciate the miracle of your body.

> **On a weekly basis,** you can spend time at a park for a bike ride or picnic; grow veggies or flowers in your garden, a large container, or a neighborhood shared pea patch; or go on a day hike.

> **On a seasonal or yearly basis,** you can celebrate nature's bounty by picking berries in summer, kicking

leaves in the fall, making snow angels in the winter, and gathering spring flowers; celebrate the holidays as they connect to the changes of the year (the winter solstice around Christmas, spring equinox near Easter, fall equinox near the Jewish New Year and Pagan holidays throughout the year); or spend part of your vacation in nature.

On a whenever basis, you can explore the patterns of nature, such as the spirals of sea shells and sunflowers; plant a seed and marvel at the miracle of its germination; and identify birds, stars, types of trees, bugs, or rocks.

Beauty

When I asked Dr. Joan Borysenko, author of *It's Not the End of the World: Developing Resilience in Times of Change*, what makes the brain work better, she said, "Beauty allows me to focus." Biophilia experts go one step further and say we can connect to nature through beauty. Beautiful places *feel* good, they say, because they help our brains resonate with the love of nature.

Think about an indoor space that makes you feel good. These features of biophilic architecture may be part of that space:

Prospect/view (an ability to see into the distance): windows or bright walls; the ability to get a long view—naturally or with mirrors; horizon and sky imagery.

Refuge (a sense of shelter where you can rest the body and mind): screens, varied light levels, penetrable surfaces for enclosure and for keeping views out, a canopy effect produced by lowered or darkened ceilings.

Water: fountains and aquariums; glimmering or reflective surfaces; symbols of water, such as seascapes, pictures of boats, and vases.

Biodiversity: varied vegetation (plants ranging from large ficus trees to small cactus and flowers), windows to incorporate nature views, outdoor natural areas, animals or images/sculptures of animals.

Sensory variety: changes and variety in color, temperature, movement (including air movement and mobiles), textures, and light.

Biomimicry (replicating nature's designs): using natural geometry, forms, and textures; fractal patterns (similar, but not identical features, like leaves on a tree) in quilts, mosaics, and even displayed collections.

Playfulness: objects, artifacts, and spaces that surprise and amuse.

Enticement (complexity that reveals itself over time): anything that encourages exploration; surfaces that gradually open.[295]

For a biophilic boost, you can incorporate any of these features into your home or office.

"It is becoming increasingly well demonstrated that biophilic elements have real, measurable benefits on productivity, emotional well-being, stress reduction, learning, and healing," says recognized architect Alex Wilson.

Biophilia and Your Body

The connection to nature is not only all around you, but also inside you, as you see, eat, sneeze, breathe, drive, poop, flirt, birth, read, and age. Your body is part of the natural planet, just like that golden zinnia in your yard or the emperor penguin in the Antarctic.

This excerpt from the famous prose poem *Desiderata* by Max Ehrmann reflects that view: "Be gentle with yourself. You are a child of the universe, no less than the trees and the stars; you have a right to be here. And whether or not it is clear to you, no doubt the universe is unfolding as it should."

It's easy to forget the miracle we're living. We live in a gotta-do culture, and our busy minds describe life, rather than experiencing it—and experiencing the body. We often see the body as the carrier of thoughts, the vehicle for earning money, or the reason we have to go to the gym or the doctor. Instead, experiencing your body as is, without doing anything, is the mysterious pathway to connecting with something bigger than yourself, says Carrie Lafferty, practitioner of Feldenkrais (sensory-movement therapy) and healing qi gong. "Your body is your subconscious mind," the level of activity just below your awareness, says neuroscientist Candace Pert.

Being in your body engages and stimulates your sensory channels for a direct contact with nature. You don't have to go anywhere, do anything, or act like anybody to experience a connection to the cycles of nature; you can do it just through your physical existence.

What do you notice when you pay attention to your body? Does your attention travel around? Does one sensation, maybe tension in your tummy, draw you in? As you focus on one area, pay attention to the images, sounds, proprioception (one's own perception of inside the body), and energies that arise. These sensations—color, movement, sound, vibration, even temperature—change over time and connect to other parts of your body.

Notice your breathing—without changing it. Most people deepen their breath as soon as they pay attention to it. Taking a deep breath is rejuvenating, but you can also notice *how* you're breathing—shallowly, exhaling with a sigh, or holding your breath—before you take a strong inhale.

Your facial expression changes your body and view of the world. Try pulling your lips down, pouting, wrinkling your brow, and hunching your shoulders and notice where your thoughts and perceptions go. See if a little smile—even an almost imperceptible one—changes your internal experience.

Softening your senses can also put you in touch with your body. When we focus on a sense—the taste of salsa, the smell of lilac, the feeling of dirty hands, or the sound of a dog barking—we usually hone in on it, closing out everything else. But softening the focus can do the opposite, expanding your senses. Notice the sounds that come and go, from the hum of the freeway to the slam of a car door to the tinnitus in your ear. Feel your whole body, from how your head rests on the spine to numbness in your shoulders to the angle of your ankles. Soften your vision to see with your peripheral (wide) focus.

This is a great meditation to do in the middle of work, especially if you've been absorbed by your computer or mind.

Love Your Expanding Brain

It's easy to forget a larger view in the day-to-day, but routines help you stay connected to a larger perspective.

Set a time and a location for **meditation** each day. You might not practice as often as you'd like, but each time you do, you'll remind your brain and body of this possibility.

Set a recurring date every morning and afternoon on your computer calendar for **stopping and breathing.** When a reminder pops up, follow its suggestion to experience your breath and body. Even one breath has a lingering effect.

If God or a higher-anything feels foreign, **pretend as if you have a connection**—even to a guardian angel. Does an image, feeling, or sound come to you? Ask to remember the connection more often for help solving a dilemma or to increase inner tranquility.

Notice what you're grateful for—not so much the stuff you have, but for the experience of life. For instance, be grateful not as much for the Audi as much as for the experience driving; not the idea of health as much as the feeling of walking; not the children, but connecting and laughing with them.

Notice nature all around you—the colors and smells of roses on a walking path, the cocoon of green in the spring, the cool air on your face, the giant trees we take for granted.

Get curious. What's in that tiny little acorn that allows it to turn into a six-story massive oak? What forces in life allow that acorn to grow? How many leaves are on that tree? How is each leaf the same, but different than the other leaves? How is each leaf connected to the others through the tree? Funny how you're just like that acorn and those leaves: connected, unique, and growing.

When Stephanie returned from vacation, she knew she had to bring something of the calm back to her life, since she couldn't bring the ocean. She created little things that added up: meditation when she remembered, pictures of herself at the ocean hung in her cube along with a few green plants, walking during her afternoon break, and connecting more to spirituality in books and friends.

Taking time to love both your brain and your body will help you feel just a little more balanced and recover your connection to something bigger. Life is still stressful, but your brain will give you enough space to let tension roll off your back a little more easily.

Chapter 14

Your Dynamic, Sparkling, Brilliant Brain

*The softest, freest, most pliable and changeful living substance is the
brain—the hardest and most iron-bound as well.*

Charlotte Perkins Gilman, author

Now that you've reached the end of this book, how do you feel about
your brain? If you picked up this book because something wasn't
quite working, did you discover what you'd like to change? Or maybe
you read this book "just because." Did something particular strike a
chord, light a spark, or touch your heart?

Perhaps you're more aware of your brain's response to hormone
fluctuations now. Or you want to spend extra time outside, eat more
greens, move more, join an improv class, purge toxic cosmetics, or
become more creative. Maybe what you *really* want is to let go of
stress and stop worrying about all the things you're not doing, doing,
doing from morning to night.

Well, however you approach it, you're taking time to make peace
with your dynamic, sparkling, brilliant womanly brain.

You don't need to put on your Superwoman cape and leap tall
changes in a single bound. Trying to make huge changes, especially
lots of them all at once, leads to inconsistency, frustration, and disappointment. And you don't need more of that.

Instead, look for the *smallest* thing that you can easily do and create
a habit. Habits use your whole brain, body, and mind—both conscious
and unconscious, to move you where you want to go. On top of that,
when you create a new habit, you not only stimulate existing neurological paths, but you also excite new brain cells so much, they can
jump old trains of thought onto new, innovative tracks.[296]

If you want to create a new helpful habit—say taking a thousand more steps a day, losing a thousand ounces (sixty-two pounds), or eating a thousand more bites of vegetables in a month (three or four carrots a day)—take the smallest possible first step, one that seems almost inconsequential. That tiny little movement will allow you to embrace success.

Recognizing exactly what a small step is can be tricky. So try the following technique based on the book *One Small Step Can Change Your Life* by Robert Maurer.

Ask yourself, "What small, trivial step can I take that could help my brain be at its best?"

"Lose weight," you might respond. A good goal, but not a small step. So ask the same question again.

"Eat less," you could answer this time. That's getting a little more specific, but it's still too big. Keep going: "What small, trivial step can I take that could help my brain be at its best?"

"Stop eating doughnuts, especially at work." You're getting more specific, but if skipping the doughnuts were an easy step, you would have done it by now. You want a step so small and easy that you can *guarantee* you'll do it every day.

What about this? For the next month, you'll throw away the first bite of a doughnut before you eat it. (Tossing out the last bite can be pretty hard.)

How does this small step help? You're making a conscious choice to eat less and learning how to start portion control. Maybe the following month you'll throw away two bites, until eventually you're eating only one bite or no doughnuts. You've learned your life works without them and your brain works better too.

Other small-step ideas:

- If you want to exercise more, try marching in front of your couch for one TV commercial a night. When you're ready for the next small step, march for two commercials and then expand to the whole commercial break.

- To exercise more and get outdoors, start by walking past three houses on your block and then back home. Add another house when you feel it is time.

- If you want to drink more water, put a pitcher on your desk. Even the empty one will remind you that your body and brain like water.

- Want to meditate more? Close your eyes and count three breaths a day. That's it. The habit will grow when you're ready.

Reminding yourself of the purpose or goal—why are you doing this?—also helps solidify a habit.[297]

The purpose of doing something isn't because you *should* or because you've been doing something *wrong*. The purpose is to increase your awareness of your brain, to create a powerful partnership. If you support your brain first, it will happily follow your lead.

Remember, everything your brain likes, your body likes too:

- Movement;

- Healthy food;

- A healthy environment;

- Connection with others;

- Stillness, rest, and sleep;

- Experiencing spirituality or something bigger;

- Hydration;

- Learning and play;

- Relaxation and stress reduction.

Supporting your brain amps up the resources you already have for creating happier, stress-free days. Then you can relish being a conscious woman who is alive—really living life—right now, right here.

Even with all the daily challenges that are yours to meet, you now know life's recipe for health and wellness: love your brain by keeping it fit, and love yourself by remembering you're worth it. Every small step you take causes your brain to whisper, "I love you too! And thanks."

Notes

1   Dan Knowles, "Most Americans Totally Stressed Out, Study Finds," AOL News article, November 10, 2010. *www.aolnews.com/2010/11/10/most-americans-totally-stressed-out-study-finds/*.

2   Quotes, Isaac Asimov, Neuroscience for Kids. And Alexis Madrigal, "Mapping the Most Complex Structure in the Universe:Your Brain," *Wired,* January, 24, 2008. *wired.com/science/discoveries/news/2008/01/connectomics.*

3   Henrietta C. Leiner and Alan L. Leiner, "The Treasure at the Bottom of the Brain," New Horizons for Learning website, "News from the Neurosciences" article, September, 1997. *www.marthalakecov.org/~building/neuro/leiner.htm.*

4   "Brain Geography (Hot Science)," an episode of the TV show Nova, air date October 7, 1997. *www.pbs.org/wgbh/nova/coma/geography/photos.html.*

5   "Telepathy is inherited in the human brain," Balkans.com Business News, February 8, 2011. *www.balkans.com/print-news.php? uniquenumber=92772.*

6   Chris Talbot, "Brain More Complex Than Previously Thought, Research Reveals," World Socialist, December 3, 2010. *www.wsws.org/articles/2010/dec2010/brai-d03.shtml.*

7   Ibid.

8   Ibid.

9   Leiner and Leiner.

10   Elizabeth Armstrong Moore, "Human Brain Has More Switches Than All Computers on Earth," CNET News, November 17, 2010. *news.cnet.com/8301-27083_3-20023112-247.html.*

11   Jeremy Coplan, "Update on Neurogenesis Research and Implications for Psychiatric Disorders," *Basic and Clinical Neuroscience Lectures,* Columbia University, February 10, 2006. *neuroscienceupdate.cumc.columbia.edu/popups/transcript_coplan.html.*

12   Eric H. Chudler, "Do We Use Only 10% of Our Brains?" Neuroscience for Kids, University of Washington, 2011. *faculty.washington.edu/chudler/tenper.html.*

13   Coplan, "Update on Neurogenesis."

14   "When Does Your Brain Function Peak?" ThirdAge.com., March 23, 2009. *www.thirdage.com/brain-fitness/when-does-your-brain-function-peak.*

15   K.Warner Schaie, "'When does age-related cognitive decline begin?' Salthouse again reifies the 'cross-sectional fallacy.'" *Pub Med Central,* National Institutes of Health, February 23, 2009. *www.ncbi.nlm.nih.gov/pmc/articles/PMC2680669/.*

16   Marcella Bombardieri, "Summer's remarks on women draw fire," *Boston.com,* January 17, 2005. *Boston.com/news/local/articles/2005/01/17/summers_remarks_on_women_draw_fire.*

17   Cordelia Fine, *Delusions of Gender: How Our Minds, Society, and Neurosexism Create Difference* (New York: W. W. Norton & Company, 2010).

18   Lise Eliot, *Pink Brain, Blue Brain: How Small Differences Grow Into Troublesome Gaps—And What We Can Do About It* (Chicago: Houghton Mifflin Harcourt, 2009).

19   Chudler, Neuroscience for Kids website.

20   Donald Pfaff, *Man and Woman: An Inside Story* (New York: Oxford University Press, 2010), 13.

21   Ibid., 9.

22   Robert M Sapolsky, *The Trouble With Testosterone: And Other Essays on the Biology of the Human Predicament* (New York: Scribner, 1998).

23   Judith Shulevitz, "Rethinking Testosterone," Slate, April 7, 2000. *www.slate.com/toolbar.aspx?action=print&id=1005049.*

24   "Testosterone Does Not Induce Aggression, Study Shows," *Science Daily,* December 9, 2009. *www.sciencedaily.com/releases/2009/12/091208132241.htm.*

25   Marla Paul, "Why Estrogen Makes You Smarter," News Center, Northwestern University, November 17, 2010. *www.northwestern.edu/newscenter/stories/2010/11/estrogen-makes-you-smarter.html.*

26   "The Hormone Connection to Women's Mental Health," *The Health,* September 12, 2010. *www.the-health.net/the-hormone-connection-to-womens-mental-health.html.*

27   Jeffrey Norris, "Estrogen Plays Key Role in Male Brain Development," University of California at San Francisco, October 1, 2009. *www.ucsf.edu/news/2009/10/8199/estrogen-plays-key-role-male-brain-development.*

28   "Estrogen and Women's Emotions," Web MD, June 19, 2011. *women.webmd.com/estrogen-and-womens-emotions.*

29   Ibid.

30   Demetria Jackson, "Effects of Progestin on the Body," eHow Health, *www.ehow.com/about_5232381_effects-progestin-body.html#ixzz1HCbQDDa9.*

31   Larry Ray Palmer, "Signs & Symptoms of Low Progesterone in Women," eHow Health*, www.ehow.com/about_5392741_signs-symptoms-low-progesterone-women.html#ixzz1HCcPomOL.*

32   Donald Stein, "Progesterone—It's more than a sex hormone," *Emory University Sound Science,* podcast and related webpage, October 2009. *whsc.emory.edu/soundscience/2009/stein.html.*

33   O. C. Schultheiss, M. M. Wirth, and S. J. Stanton, "Effects of Affiliation and Power Motivation Arousal on Salivary Progesterone and Testosterone," *Hormones and Behavior* 46, no. 5 (December 2004), 592–599.

34   M. G. Kibria, "List of Human Hormones," *MedicBD Health, www.health.medicbd.com/wiki/List_of_human_hormones.*

35   Sally Law, "Dads, Too, Get Hormone Boost While Caring for Baby," *Live Science, TechMediaNetwork.com,* October 5, 2010. *www.livescience.com/10784-dads-hormone-boost-caring-baby.html.*

36   Marianne J. Legato, *Why Men Never Remember and Women Never Forget.* New York: Rodale Books, 2005.

37   "Oxytocin and Women," *Oxytocin Accelerator, oxytocinaccelerator.com/oxytocin-and-woman.*

38   David S. Cooper, "Graves' Disease," *Womenshealth.gov,* May 18, 2010. *www.womenshealth.gov/faq/graves-disease.cfm.*

39   Kresimira Milas and Kamiah A Walker, "Hyperthyroidism Symptoms," Endocrine Web, October 13, 2010. *www.endocrineweb.com/conditions/hyperthyroidism/hyperthyroidism-symptoms.*

40   Cooper, "Graves' Disease."

41   T. L. Dellovade, Y. S. Zhu, L. Krey, D. W. Pfaff, "Thyroid Hormone and Estrogen Interact to Regulate Behavior," *Proceedings of the National Academies of Sciences* 93, no. 22 (October 29, 1996), 12581–12586. *www.ncbi.nlm.nih.gov/pmc/articles/PMC38035/*.

42   Gunjan Tykodi, personal interview. March 10, 2011.

43   Flux, *stereopsis.com/flux/*.

44   Steven D. Ehrlich, "Melatonin," University of Maryland Medical Center, April–May, 2009. *www.umm.edu/altmed/articles/melatonin-000315.htm*.

45   Ibid.

46   "Man flu DOES exist—study suggests half of men exaggerate cold symptoms," Mail Online, June 8, 2010. *www.dailymail.co.uk/health/article-1284927/Man-flu-DOES-exist--study-suggests-half-men-exaggerate-cold-symptoms.html*.

47   Pfaff, *Man and Woman*, 132.

48   Linda Lewis Alexander, Judith Larosa, William James Alexander, *New Dimensions in Women's Health,* 5th edition (Sudbury, MA: Jones & Bartlett, 2009).

49   James, "The Enemy Within—Autoimmune Disorder," *Ygoy: Health & Lifestyle Updates,* October 18, 2009, *www.ygoy.com/index.php/the-enemy-within-our-own-body---autoimmune-disorder/*.

50   Alexander, Larosa, Alexander.

51   S. Ansar Ahmed, W. J. Penhale, and N. Talal, "Sex hormones, immune responses, and autoimmune diseases. Mechanisms of sex hormone action," *American Journal of Pathology* 121, no. 3 (December 1985), 531–551. *www.ncbi.nlm.nih.gov/pubmed/3907369*.

52   A. H. W. M. Schuurs and H. A. M. Verheul, "Sex Hormones and Autoimmune Disease," *Rheumatology* 28 (1989), 59–61. *rheumatology.oxfordjournals.org/content/XXVIII/suppl_1/59.abstract*.

53   Greg Nalbandian and Susan Kovats, "Estrogen, Immunity & Autoimmune Disease," Beckman Research Institute.

December 8, 2004, *www.benthamscience.com/cmciema/sample/cmciema5-1/0010P.pdf*.

54   Marcelle Pick, "Fatigue & Insomnia," *Women to Women,* April 20, 2011, article online. *www.womentowomen.com/fatigueandstress/insomnia.aspx*. And Kenneth L. Lichstein, H. Heith Durrence, Brant W. Riedel, and Daniel J. Taylor, *Epidemiology of Sleep: Age, Gender, and Ethnicity* (Psychology Press, 2004), 155.

55   "Child Sexual Abuse," *The National Center for Victims of Crime,* 2008, webpage content. *www.ncvc.org/ncvc/main.aspx?dbName=DocumentViewer&DocumentID=32315*.

56   "Seasonal Affective Disorder (SAD)," *Mental Health America,* February 2002, *www.nmha.org/go/sad*.

57   Humphries, Courtney. "Vitamin D and seasonal affective disorder." *The Boston Globe.* December 14, 2009. *www.boston.com/news/health/articles/2009/12/14/vitamin_d_and_seasonal_affective_disorder/*.

58   M. Said. "Seasonal Affective Disorders." Priory.com. Priory Lodge Education Ltd, January, 2001. *priory.com/psych/sad.htm*.

59   Carolyn Bernstein and Elaine McArdle, *The Migraine Brain: Your Breakthrough Guide to Fewer Headaches, Better Health* (New York: Free Press, 2008).

60   Ibid.

61   Christian Nordqvist, "Tinted Lenses Relieve Migraine Symptoms, Neurological Proof," *Medical News Today,* May 25, 2011. *www.medicalnewstoday.com/articles/226465.php.*

62   "The Brain Chemistry of Depression—Stress Hormones," Psycheducation.org. *www.psycheducation.org/mechanism/stress%20hormone%20intro.htm.*

63   Karen J. Berkley, Steven S. Zalcman, and Viviana R. Simon, "Sex and gender differences in pain and inflammation: a rapidly maturing field," *American Journal of Physiology—Regulatory, Integrative and Comparative* 291, no. 2 (August 2006), R241–R244. *ajpregu.physiology.org/content/291/2/R241.full.*

64   Pfaff, *Man and Woman.*

65   A. K. Sharma, V. P. Gupta, H. Bhardwaj, H. Prakash, R. Gupta, "High Prevalence of Hypertension in the Desert-Based Rural Population of Rajasthan," *South Asian Journal of Preventive Cardiology* 7, no. 2 (April–June 2003). *www.sajpc.org/vol7/vol7_2/highprevalence.htm.*

66   "Understanding & Navigating the Maternity Care System: Hormones Driving Labor and Birth," *Childbirth Connection,* April 10, 2011. *www.childbirthconnection.org/article.asp?ck=10184.*

67   Viktoria Carrella, "Symptoms of Estrogen Loss," *eHow Health. www.ehow.com/about_5125674_symptoms-estrogen-loss.html#ixzz15o5Rbwvo.*

68   Marcelle Pick, "Menopause & Perimenopause: Estrogen dominance—is it real?" *Women to Women,* June 2, 2001, *www.womentowomen.com/menopause/estrogendominance.aspx.*

69   "Estrogen Multiplies Synapses Between Neurons." Softpedia. April 11, 2011. *news.softpedia.com/news/Estrogen-Multiplies-Synapses-Between-Neurons-167267.shtml.*

70   A. S. Nowacek and D. R. Sengelaub, "Estrogenic support of motoneuron dendritic growth via the neuromuscular periphery in a sexually dimorphic motor system," *Journal of Neurobiology* 66, no. 9 (August 2006), 962–976. *www.ncbi.nlm.nih.gov/pubmed/16779828.*

71   Estrogen has many positive effects on neural tissue in experimental model systems, including stimulation of neurite growth and neurotransmitter synthesis and protection against diverse types of neural injury.

72   "Birth Control Controlling Your Sex Drive?" Epigee Women's Health, 2011. *www.epigee.org/guide/pill_sex.html.*

73   Deborah Sichel and Jeanne Watson Driscoll, *Women's Moods, Women's Minds: What Every Woman Must Know About Hormones, the Brain, and Emotional Health* (New York: William Morrow, 1999).

74   "Menopause and HRT: Hormones and the Menstrual Cycle," *Holistic online.com,* 2002. *www.holisticonline.com/remedies/hrt/hrt_menstr_hormone.htm.*

75   Marcy Holmes, "PMS and PMDD—natural solutions," *Women to Women,* May 18, 2011. *www.womentowomen.com/menstruation/understandingpmsandpmdd.aspx.*

76   Richard Karel, "Hormones and Benzodiazepines: PMS, Postpartum Depression, Sedative Withdrawal Believed to Have Common Brain-Receptor Link," *Benzodiazepine Withdrawal Support, www.benzosupport.org/Hormones%20and%20benzo%20diazepines.htm.* And Jennifer Warner, "Menstrual Cycle May Alter Brain Chemistry," *FoxNews.com,* May 15, 2005. *www.foxnews.com/story/0,2933,156703,00.html.*

77   Chris Sherwood, "How Does Midol Work?" *eHow Health*. *www.ehow.com/how-does_5207451_midol-work_.html#ixzz1HxtgQbiR*.

78   Bruce S. McEwen and M. Kalia, "The role of corticosteroids and stress in chronic pain conditions," *Metabolism* 59 Supplement (October 2010), S9–15. *www.ncbi.nlm.nih.gov/pubmed/20837196*.

79   T. C. Frank, G. L. Kim, A. Krzemien, D. A. Van Vugt, "Effect of menstrual cycle phase on corticolimbic brain activation by visual food cues," *Brain Research* 1363 (December 2, 2010), 81–92. *www.ncbi.nlm.nih.gov/pubmed/20920491*.

80   Gary Wenk, "Chocolate: The Good, the Bad and the Angry," *Psychology Today,* November 10, 2010. *www.psychologytoday.com/blog/your-brain-food/201011/chocolate-the-good-the-bad-and-the-angry*.

81   "PMS & PMDD," *MGH Center for Women's Mental Health, www.womensmentalhealth.org/specialty-clinics/pms-and-pmdd/*.

82   Ibid.

83   John R. Lee, "Facts About PMS," The Official Site of John R. Lee, M.D., *www.johnleemd.com/store/pms_facts.html*.

84   "Premenstrual dysphoric disorder—Overview," *University of Maryland Medical Center, www.umm.edu/ency/article/007193.htm*.

85   Steven D. Ehrlich, "Premenstrual Syndrome," *University of Maryland Medical Center,* June 27, 2010, *www.umm.edu/altmed/articles/premenstrual-syndrome-000132.htm*.

86   "Study Links Smoking to PMS in Women," *NBC DFW,* July 17, 2009, *www.nbcdfw.com/news/health/Smoking-Linked-to-PMS-in-Women.html*.

87   "An Optimum Diet to manage PMS," *Women Fitness.net, www.womenfitness.net/manage-pms.htm*.

88   "Study Shows Low-Fat Diet Reduces Disabling Cramps and PMS," *News and Media Center,* media advisory from the Physicians Committee for Responsible Medicine, January 31, 2000. *www.pcrm.org/news/research000131.html*.

89   Sarah Terry, "Natural Relief from PMS," *livestrong.com,* July 10, 2010. *www.livestrong.com/article/170631-natural-relief-from-pms/#ixzz15tGza7ll*.

90   "Magnesium and PMS," Natural Calm Magnesium Supplements (product website). *www.calmnatural.com/magnesium-and-pms*.

91   Ehrlich, "Premenstrual Syndrome."

92   August Mclaughlin, "Fish Oil for PMS," *livestrong.com,* June 17, 2010. *www.livestrong.com/article/151293-fish-oil-for-pms/#ixzz1I3NfhkZn*.

93   "Acupuncture and PMT," *The London Acupuncture Space. www.londonacupuncturespace.com/acupuncture-pmspmt-london.htm*.

94   "Placebos Work—Even Without Deception," *ScienceDaily,* December 23, 2010. *www.sciencedaily.com/releases/2010/12/01222173033.htm*.

95   Sichel and Driscoll.

96   Sichel and Driscoll, 153.

97   "Memory Decreases During Pregnancy," Wayne State University School of Medicine, article online. *www.med.wayne.edu/Scribe/scribe97-98/scribew98/memory.htm*.

98   Sichel and Driscoll, xii.

99   "What is Perimenopause?" *ThirdAge.com,* August 9, 2009. *www.thirdage.com/menopause/what-is-perimenopause#ixzz16XDFSilw*.

100 "Perimenopause: Rocky road to menopause," Harvard Heath Publications. Harvard University, Aug. 2005, *www.health.harvard.edu/newsweek/Perimenopause_Rocky_road_to_menopause.htm.*

101 Christiane Northrup, *Women's Bodies, Women's Wisdom* (New York: Bantam, 2002).

102 Bruce S. McEwen, "The Molecular and Neuroanatomical Basis for Estrogen Effects in the Central Nervous System," *The Journal of Clinical Endocrinology & Metabolism* 84, no. 6 (1999): 1790–1797. *jcem.endojournals.org/content/84/6/1790.full.pdf+html?sid=7156e8b4-4a44-476e-996b-e2bc7801cc00.*

103 J. E. Brody, "Hormone replacement: Weighing risks and benefits," *The New York Times,* February 1, 2000.

104 Kristine Yaffe, "Hormone Therapy and the Brain: Déja Vu All Over Again?" (editorial), *Journal of the American Medical Association* 289, no. 20 (2003), 2717–2719. *jama.ama-assn.org/content/289/20/2717.short.*

105 Elaine Stretch, personal interview, February 26, 2011.

106 Pam Harrison, "No increased stroke risk with low-dose HRT patch?" *Theheart.org,* June 7, 2010. *www.theheart.org/article/1086039.do.*

107 Brian Hayes, "From Motricity to Mentality," *American Scientist,* July 2001. *www.americanscientist.org/bookshelf/pub/from-motricity-to-mentality.*

108 Fernando Pagés Ruiz, "What Is Consciousness?" *Yoga Journal,* September–October 2001, 104–174.

109 Ibid.

110 Christine DiMaria, "Why Does Exercise Help Your Brain?" *livestrong.com,* June 14, 2011. *www.livestrong.com/article/382203-why-does-exercise-help-your-brain/.*

111 James Levine, "Staffing Firm Salo Becomes America's First 'Office of the Future' in Mayo Clinic Study Measuring Impact of Movement on Weight & Wellness," *Oberon,* August 2, 2008.

112 John J. Ratey and Eric Hagerman. *Spark: The Revolutionary New Science of Exercise and the Brain* (New York: Little, Brown and Company, 2008).

113 Ibid., 5.

114 Ibid., 40.

115 "Exercising the Brain," University of New South Wales news release, July 14, 2010. *www.unsw.edu.au/news/pad/articles/2010/jul/Morris_exercise.html.*

116 Ratey. 45.

117 Ibid., 51.

118 Ibid., 92.

119 Ibid., 107–108.

120 Ibid., 117, 121.

121 Ibid., 158.

122 Ibid., 177, 178.

123 Ibid., 209.

124 Ibid., 223.

125 Caroline Wilbert, "Are Americans Backing Off Exercise?" WebMD, January 21, 2010. *www.webmd.com/fitness-exercise/news/20100121/are-americans-backing-off-exercise.*

126 "Stress: Your brain and body," *Your Amazing Brain*. *www.youramazingbrain.org/brainchanges/stressbrain.htm*.

137 Sara Mahoney, "Exercise & Cortisol Levels," *livestrong.com,* March 18, 2011. *www.livestrong.com/article/86687-exercise-cortisol-levels/#ixzz1IzbhsksA*.

128 William C. Dement and Christopher Vaughan, *The Promise of Sleep: A Pioneer in Sleep Medicine Explores the Vital Connection Between Health, Happiness, and a Good Night's Sleep* (New York: Dell, 2000).

129 Eric H. Chudler, "Brain Tries To Help After Sleep Deprivation," *Neuroscience For Kids,* February 25, 2000. *faculty.washington.edu/chudler/sleepc.html*.

130 "Impact of Sleep Deprivation On Brain Functioning Different Than Previously Thought," *Medical News Today,* February 11, 2010.

131 Caroline Cassels, "Overweight and Obesity Linked to Lower Brain Volume," Medscape News, August 28, 2009. *www.medscape.com/viewarticle/708090*.

132 "Effects of Sleep Deprivation," *Shift-your-consciousness.com*. *www.shift-your-consciousness.com/effects-of-sleep-deprivation.html*.

133 "Sex and the Brain," *Fit Brains,* August 18, 2008. *www.fitbrains.com/blog/2008/08/18/sex-and-the-brain/*.

134 Matthew Edlund, MD, "Can Sex Grow My Brain?" *Psychology Today*. Sussex Directories. Inc., August 5, 2010. *www.psychologytoday.com/blog/the-power-rest/201008/can-sex-grow-my-brain*.

135 Mark Henderson, "Women fall into 'trance' during orgasm," *The Times,* June 20, 2005. *www.timesonline.co.uk/tol/life_and_style/health/article535521.ece*.

136 Tania Romero, "Neurobiology of Human Sexuality," Bryn Mawr College research paper, April 23, 2002. *serendip.brynmawr.edu/bb/neuro/neuro02/web2/tromero.html*.

137 Mark Stibich, "Top 10 Sex Tips for the Older Woman," *About.com,* January 24, 2009. *longevity.about.com/od/healthyagingandlongevity/tp/sex_tips_women.htm*.

138 Andrew Newberg and Mark Robert Waldman, *How God Changes Your Brain: Breakthrough Findings from a Leading Neuroscientist* (New York: Ballantine Books, 2010).

139 "Endorphin and enkephalin," *Medical Discoveries*. *www.discoveriesinmedicine.com/Com-En/Endorphin-and-Enkephalin.html*.

140 Mary Payne Bennett and Cecile Lengacher. "Humor and Laughter May Influence Health: II. Complementary Therapies and Humor in a Clinical Population." PubMed Central. U.S. National Library of Medicine, February 20, 2006. *www.ncbi.nlm.nih.gov/pmc/articles/pmc1475938/*.

141 Kareem J. Johnson, Christian E. Waugh, and Barbara L. Fredrickson, "Smile to see the forest: Facially expressed positive emotions broaden cognition," *Cognition & Emotion* 24, no. 2 (2010) 299–321.

142 "Smiling," *The Oxford Companion to the Body* (New York: Oxford University Press, 2001, 2003). Referenced on Answers.com. *www.answers.com/topic/smiling-2*.

143 The Franklin Institute, "How Your Brain Responds to Stress," *Resources for Science Learning,* 2004. *www.fi.edu/learn/brain/stress.html*.

144 Libby Pelham, "Health Advice: Football Concussion Take Their Toll," *Families.com,* October 3, 2010. *health.families.com/blog/football-concussion-take-their-toll*.

145 "Head Injuries in Football," *New York Times,* October 21, 2010. *topics.nytimes.com/top/reference/timestopics/subjects/f/football/head_injuries/index.html*.

146 "The Top 5 Causes of Head Injuries and How to Avoid Them," *SixWise.com,* *www.sixwise.com/newsletters/05/09/28/the-top-5-causes-of-head-injuries-and-how-to-avoid-them.htm.*

147 "Helmet Related Statistics from Many Sources," Bicycle Helmet Safety Institute, *www.helmets.org/stats.htm.*

148 Rick Nauert, "Researchers Look to Define Wisdom," *PsychCentral,* May 10, 2010. *psychcentral.com/news/2010/05/10/researchers-look-to-define-wisdom/13658.html.*

149 Dov Michaeli, "Brain Plasticity: Is There a Limit?" *The Doctor Weighs In,* March 3, 2011. *www.thedoctorweighsin.com/brain-plasticity-is-there-a-limit/.*

150 Michael Merzenich, "About Brain Plasticity," On the Brain, April 16, 2008. *merzenich.positscience.com/?page_id=143.*

151 Keay Davidson, "Brain is built to forget, research says," *SF Gate,* January 9, 2004. *www.sfgate.com/cgi-bin/article.cgi?f=/c/a/2004/01/09/MNG6C46SQ01.DTL&ao =2#ixzz18gL6M82Z.*

152 Emma S. McDonald, "More Bang for Your Buck: Movement and Learning," *Inspiring Teachers,* January 14, 2010. *inspiringteachers.blogspot.com/2010/01/more-bang-for-your-buck-movement-and.html.*

153 "Memorizing Through Association," *Rememberg.com,* 2010. *www.rememberg.com/ Mnemonic-Systems/Z-Association--Memorizing-through-Association.*

154 William R. Klemm, "Music Training Helps Learning & Memory," July 31, 2010. *Psychology Today, www.psychologytoday.com/blog/memory-medic/201007/music-training-helps-learning-memory.*

155 Ibid.

156 Michael Gazzaniga, Carolyn Asbury, and Barbara Rich, editors. "Learning, Arts, and the Brain," The Dana Foundation. *www.dana.org/uploadedfiles/news_ and_publications/special_publications/learning,%20arts%20and%20the%20brain_ artsandcognition_compl.pdf.*

157 Michael I. Posner, "How Arts Training Improves Attention and Cognition," The Dana Foundation, September 14, 2009. *www.creativityaustralia.com.au/docs/The-Dana-Foundation-How-Arts-Training-Improves-Attention-and-Cognition.pdf.*

158 Stuart L. Brown and Christopher C. Vaughan. *Play: How It Shapes the Brain, Opens the Imagination, and Invigorates the Soul.* New York: Avery, 2010. 29.

159 Nancy Shute, "10 Reasons Play Can Make You Healthy, Happy, and More Productive," *U.S. News & World Report: Health,* March 9. 2009. *health.usnews.com/ health-news/family-health/childrens-health/articles/2009/03/09/10-reasons-play-can-make-you-healthy-happy-and-more-productive.html.*

160 "Play Science—The Patterns of Play." The National Institute for Play. *www. nifplay.org/states_play.html.*

161 Richard Restak, *Mozart's Brain and the Fighter Pilot: Unleashing Your Brain's Potential.* New York: Three Rivers Press, 2002.

162 Howard Gardner, "Multiple Intelligences After Twenty Years." Paper presented at the American Educational Research Association, Chicago, Illinois, April 21, 2003. *www.pz.harvard.edu/PIs/HG_MI_after_20_years.pdf.*

163 "Top 10 Electronic Reminder Services." Top Web Resources. April 15, 2009. *www.iyiz.com/top-10-electronic-reminder-services/.*

164 Nancy C. Andreasen, *The Creating Brain: The Neuroscience of Genius.* New York: Dana, 2005. 73.

165 "Mirror Therapy for Phantom Limb Pain," *The New England Journal of Medicine* 357 (November 22, 2007), 2206–2207. *www.nejm.org/doi/full/10.1056/NEJMc071927.*

166 Mo, "Ramachandran on consciousness, mirror neurons & phantom limb syndrome," October 5, 2007. From the blog "Neurophilosophy." *neurophilosophy.wordpress.com/2006/10/05/ramachandran-on-concsiousness-mirror-neurons-phantom-limb-sydrome/.*

167 Alfred Adler, *What Life Should Mean to You* (First published in 1931), chapter 2.

168 "Mind," Dictionary.com. *dictionary.reference.com/browse/mind.*

169 Molly Gordon, "Psst! Your Body Would Like a Word with You: How Tuning Into Your Body Can Help Your Biz," March 20, 2009. Blog entry on *Shaboom Inc., shaboominc.com/blog/archives/psst_your_body_would_like_a_word_with_you_how_tuning_into_your_body_can_help_your_biz.html.*

170 Jaktraks, "The Importance of Emotions: Are Emotions More Trouble Than They're Worth?" *Squidoo* (Topics, Healthy Living, Mental Health, Personal Development). *www.squidoo.com/needemotions.*

171 Paul Mason, "Role of Emotions in Brain Function," August 26, 2008. From the blog "Neuroanthropology." *neuroanthropology.net/2008/08/26/role-of-emotions-in-brain-function/.*

172 Om Paramapooya, "What Part of the Brain Controls Emotions?" *eHow Health,* March 28, 2011. *www.ehow.com/about_5483907_part-brain-controls-emotions.html.*

173 Ragini Michaels, "Emotions, Personality and the True Self," class presentation, February 5, 2006.

174 Ernesto A. Randolfi, "Exercise as a Stress Management Modality," Optimal Health Concepts. *www.optimalhealthconcepts.com/ExerciseStress.html.*

175 Karla Talanian, "Keeping Fit: Studies show links between exercise and mood," The Harvard Press, September 24, 2010. *www.harvardpress.com/DesktopModules/DnnForge%20-%20NewsArticles/Print.aspx?tabid=2190&tabmoduleid=7735&articleId=5749&moduleId=3353&PortalID=0&PageID=876.*

176 Jonathan Mandell, "Eating 101: First Recipe, Finally Cooked. Or: Why Many People Don't Cook," *The Faster Times,* September 9, 2009. *thefastertimes.com/eating101/2009/09/09/first-recipe-finally-cooked-or-why-many-people-dont-cook/.*

177 David Kessler, *The End of Overeating: Taking Control of the Insatiable American Appetite* (New York: Rodale Books, 2009).

178 "Fat Basics," *Fats of Life Newsletter: Research Summaries for Consumers About Healthy Fats. www.fatsoflife.com/fat-basics.php.*

179 Cherie Calbom, "The surprising truth about saturated fats." *PCC Sound Consumer,* PCC Natural Markets, February, 2006. *www.pccnaturalmarkets.com/sc/0602/sc0602-saturatedfats.html.*

180 Ibid.

181 Laura Dolson, "Trans Fat," Low Carb Diets, About.com, April 22, 2008. *lowcarbdiets.about.com/od/glossary/g/transfat.htm.*

182 "What is hydrogenation, anyway?" Trans Fat Free. *www.transfatfree.com/pages/art_hydrogenation.htm.*

183 "Know Your Fats," American Heart Association, June 14, 2011. *www.heart.org/ HEARTORG/Conditions/Cholesterol/PreventionTreatmentofHighCholesterol/Know-Your-Fats_UCM_305628_Article.jsp.*

184 "Fat Basics." (See note 178.)

185 Mary Enig and Sally Fallon. "Proven Health Benefits of Saturated Fats." Organic Natural Health. *health-report.co.uk/saturated_fats_health_benefits.htm.*

186 Jane Houlihan, "Results from tests of store-bought farmed salmon show 7 of 10 fish were so contaminated with PCBs that they raise cancer risk," Environmental Working Group, July 2003. *www.ewg.org/reports/farmedpcbs.*

187 The Chicago Health and Aging Project.

188 Keiko Unno and Minoru Hoshino, "Brain Senescence and Neurouprotective Dietary Components," *Central Nervous System Agents in Medicinal Chemistry* 7, no. 2 (2007): 109–114. *www.benthamscience.com/cmccnsa/openaccessarticles/cmccnsa7-2/0004T.pdf.*

189 S. Schmitt-Schillig, et al. "Flavonoids and the aging brain." *PubMed.gov.* U.S. National Library of Medicine, March, 2005. *www.ncbi.nlm.nih.gov/pubmed/15800383.*

190 Unno and Hoshimo, "Brain Senescence and Neuroprotective Dietary Components."

191 Michelle Micallef, "Red wine consumption increases antioxidant status and decreases oxidative stress in the circulation of both young and old humans," *Nutrition Journal* 6, no. 27 (September 24, 2007).

192 Tyson Alexander, "The Benefits of Pomegranate Juice for the Brain." livestrong.com, September 28, 2010. *www.livestrong.com/article/261199-the-benefits-of-pomegranate-juice-for-the-brain/.*

193 Veronique Casse, "Chia Seeds—Natural Super Brain Food for all Ages." Suite101, *www.suite101.com/content/chia-seeds---natural-super-brain-food-for-all-ages-a278057.*

194 "Saffron for Depression," Bastyr Center for Natural Health, 2011. *www. bastyrcenter.org/content/view/687/.*

195 The George Mateljan Foundation for the World's Healthiest Foods, "Cinnamon, Ground." The World's Healthiest Foods. *www.whfoods.com/genpage. php?tname=foodspice&dbid=68.*

196 "Daily Caffeine 'protects brain,'" BBC News, April 2, 2008. *news.bbc.co.uk/2/ hi/7326839.stm.*

197 Dharma Singh Khalsa, MD. *Brain Longevity.* New York: Grand Central Publishing, 1999, p. 265.

198 Pradeep J. Nathan, Kristy Lu, M. Gray, and C. Oliver, "The Neuropharmacology of L-Theanine (N-Ethyl-L-Glutamine) A Possible Neuroprotective and Cognitive Enhancing Agent," *Journal of Herbal Pharmacotherapy* 6, no. 2 (2006), 21–30. *informahealthcare.com/doi/abs/10.1080/J157v06n02_02.*

199 Bonnie Prescott, "Study Finds Heavy Drinking Linked to Higher Stroke Risk," January 5, 2005. Press release from the Beth Israel Deaconess Medical Center. *www. bidmc.org/News/InResearch/2005/January/StudyFindsHeavyDrinkingLinkedToHigher StrokeRisk.aspx.*

200 Julie Steenhuysen, "Feeding your brain: new benefits found in chocolate." Reuters: UK Edition, February 18, 2007. *uk.reuters.com/article/2007/02/20/health-cocoa-brain-dc-idUKN1836014620070220.*

201 Donald Hensrud, "Medical Edge Newspaper Column: Food Sources the Best Choice for Antioxidants," Mayo Clinic, June 5, 2009. *www.mayoclinic.org/medical-edge-newspaper-2009/jun-05b.html.*

202 Dori Khakpour, personal interview, March, 2008.

203 Edward Giovannucci, "Ask the Expert: Vitamin D and Chronic Disease," *Harvard School of Public Health. www.hsph.harvard.edu/nutritionsource/questions/vitamin-d-and-chronic-disease/index.html.*

204 Diane Welland, "Does Vitamin D Improve Brain Function?" *Scientific American,* November 2, 2009. *www.scientificamerican.com/article.cfm?id=does-d-make-a-difference.*

205 Dr. Mary *Eileen Stretch, ND, personal interview,* 2011.

206 National Library of Medicine, National Institutes of Health, "Boron," *MedlinePlus,* May 18, 2011. *www.nlm.nih.gov/medlineplus/druginfo/natural/894.html.*

207 Pfaff. AU: is this from *Man and Woman* or the journal article he collaborated on?

208 Steven D. Ehrlich, "Copper," *University of Maryland Medical Center,* March 20, 2009. *www.umm.edu/altmed/articles/copper-000296.htm.*

209 Steven D. Ehrlich, "Zinc," *University of Maryland Medical Center,* June 18, 2009. *www.umm.edu/altmed/articles/zinc-000344.htm.*

210 M. R. Joffres, T. Williams, B. Sabo, et al., "Environmental Sensitivities: Prevalence of Major Symptoms in a Referral Center," *The Nova Scotia Environmental Sensitivities Research Center Study, Environ Health Perspective* 109, no. 2 (2001), 161–165.

211 Richard Alleyne, "Shopping styles of men and women all down to evolution, claim scientists," *The Telegraph UK,* December 3, 2009. *www.telegraph.co.uk/science/science-news/6720150/Shopping-styles-of-men-and-women-all-down-to-evolution-claim-scientists.html.*

212 "Detox," *Buzzle.com. www.buzzle.com/articles/detoxify-and-lose-weight.html.*

213 According to the Institute for Agriculture and Trade Policy's 2006 report, "Playing Chicken: Avoiding Arsenic in Your Meat," updated June 8, 2011on their blog: *www.iatp.org/blog/201106/major-contributor-of-arsenic-in-animal-feed-halts-practice.*

214 Linda Tarr Kent, "Estrogenic Foods to Avoid," *Livestrong.com,* March 17, 2011. *www.livestrong.com/article/70189-estrogenic-foods-avoid/#ixzz1IRT0KgsX.*

215 "Bovine Growing Hormone (rGBH)," Shirley's Wellness Café, January 29, 2010. *www.shirleys-wellness-cafe.com/bgh.htm.*

216 Environmental Working Group, "EWG's Skin Deep Cosmetics Database: Nitrosamines." *www.cosmeticsdatabase.com/ingredient.php?ingred06=726336.*

217 "Dioxin poisoning," IdeaConnection. *www.ideaconnection.com/solutions/569-Dioxin-poisoning.html.*

218 Jeanie Lerche Davis, "Smoking Cigarettes Affects Brain Like Heroin," WebMD Health News, October 27, 2004. *www.webmd.com/smoking-cessation/news/20041027/smoking-cigarettes-affects-brain-like-heroin.*

219 Catharine Paddock, "Smoking Linked to Brain Damage, New Study," *Medical News Today,* June 23, 2009. *www.medicalnewstoday.com/articles/155038.php.*

220 "Why is Smoking Addictive?" *Ygoy. smoking.ygoy.com/2007/12/27/why-is-smoking-addictive/.*

221 "Effects of Smoking on the Brain," *Ygoy. smoking.ygoy.com/effects-of-smoking-on-the-brain/.*

222 Meredith Melnick, "Study: Heavy Smoking in Midlife Hikes the Risk of Alzheimer's," *Time: Healthland,* October 26, 2010. *healthland.time.com/2010/10/26/study-heavy-smoking-in-midlife-more-than-doubles-the-risk-of%C2%A0alzheimers/.*

223 Environmental Working Group, "Limit Your Exposure to Cell Phone Radiation," *Environmental Working Group,* December, 2010. *www.ewg.org/cellphone-radiation.*

224 Courtney Hutchinson, "Cell Phones Increase Brain Activity, Stir Fears," *Good Morning America,* ABC, February 20, 2011. *abcnews.go.com/Health/Wellness/cell-phone-study-cell-ups-brain-activity/story?id=12971636.*

225 Connie Thompson, "Site warns of toxins in beauty products," *Komonews.com,* May 5, 2008. *www.komonews.com/news/18680399.html.*

226 Emily Main, "Chemicals in Plastic Linked to Low IQs in Kids," *Rodale,* March 16, 2010. *www.rodale.com/phthalate-plasticizers.*

227 Evan Johnson, "Sweet Smell of Death," All Natural Health. *allnaturalhealth.us/evan_johnson_perfume_truth.htm.*

228 Ibid.

229 Radha McLean, "Soap Ingredients to Avoid," Livestrong.com, May 4, 2010. *www.livestrong.com/article/116612-soap-ingredients-avoid/.*

230 Jasmin Malik Chua, "Know Your Cosmetics Ingredients: Top Five Ingredients to Avoid," Planet Green.com, February 19, 2008. *planetgreen.discovery.com/fashion-beauty/toxic-cosmetics-ingredients.html.*

231 Ibid.

232 "Harmful Ingredients in Household Cleaning Products," Pure Zing. *www.purezing.com/living/toxins/living_toxins_harmfulhousehold.html.*

233 Audrey Kunin, "Allergic to New Clothes? Formaldehyde Finish May Be the Cause," Bottom Line Secrets, May 14, 2009. *www.bottomlinesecrets.com/article.html?article_id=48716.*

234 Ibid.

235 Raymond Singer and Dana Darby Johnson, "Recognizing Neurotoxicity," Neurotoxic Chemical Effects Information. *www.neurotox.com/documents/Recognizing_Neurotoxicity.pdf.*

236 Edward M. Hallowell, *Overloaded Circuits: Why Smart People Underperform* (Harvard Business Review OnPoint enhanced e-book, 2009).

237 Matt Richtel, "Attached to Technology and Paying a Price," *The New York Times,* June 6, 2010. *www.nytimes.com/2010/06/07/technology/07brain.html?_r=1&emc=eta1&pagewanted=all.*

238 Paul E. Dux, et al., "Training Improves Multitasking Performance by Increasing the Speed of Information Processing in Human Prefrontal Cortex," *Neuron* 63 (July 16, 2009), 127–138. *www.psy.vanderbilt.edu/faculty/marois/Publications/Dux_et_al-2009.pdf.*

239 Ibid.

240 Patricia M. Greenfield, "Technology and Informal Education: What Is Taught, What Is Learned," *Science* 323, no. 69 (January 2, 2009). *a.parsons.edu/~loretta/assessment_archive/science/Greenfield.pdf.*

241 Linda Stone, "Continuous Partial Attention," blog entry at Linda Stone. *lindastone.net/qa/continuous-partial-attention/.*

242 "Digital Information Overload," Youth and Media. *youthandmedia.org/wiki/ Digital_Information_Overload.*

243 Alorie Gilbert, "Newsmaker: Why Can't You Pay Attention Anymore?" CNET News, March 28, 2005. *news.cnet.com/Why-cant-you-pay-attention-anymore/2008-1022_3-5637632.html#ixzz19UFCllQF.*

244 Nicholas Carr. "Is Google Making Us Stupid?" *The Atlantic.* July–August, 2008. *www.theatlantic.com/magazine/archive/2008/07/is-google-making-us-stupid/6868/.*

245 Norman Doidge, *The Brain That Changes Itself: Stories of Personal Triumph from the Frontiers of Brain Science* (New York: Viking Adult, 2007), 309.

246 Lea Goldman, "This Is Your Brain on Clicks," Forbes.com. *members.forbes.com/ forbes/2005/0509/054.html, May 9, 2005.*

247 "Stay on Target," *The Economist,* June 10, 2010. *www.economist.com/node/ 16295664.*

248 Nicholas Carr, "First Steps to Digital Detox," *The New York Times,* June 7, 2010. *roomfordebate.blogs.nytimes.com/2010/06/07/first-steps-to-digital-detox/.*

249 Brandon Keim, "Good Connection Really Does Lead to Mind Meld," *Wired,* July 26, 2010. *www.wired.com/wiredscience/2010/07/mind-meshing/.*

250 Eddie Harmon-Jones and Piotr Winkielman, editors, *Social Neuroscience: Integrating Biological and Psychological Explanations of Social Behavior* (New York: The Guilford Press, 2007).

251 Melissa J. Moore and Mario P. Casa de Calvo, "Social Connectivity: How the Brain Helps to Shape Interactions," *Journal of Scientific Psychology,* September, 2008. *psyencelab.com/archive.html.*

252 Todd Hargrove, "Mirror Neurons—Can You Get Better at Sports by Just Watching?" April 1, 2010, blog entry on "Better Movement." *toddhargrove.wordpress. com/2010/04/01/mirror-neurons-can-you-get-better-at-sports-by-just-watching/.*

253 "15 Practices to Deepen Human Connection and Engagement Online," *The Brain Alchemist,* July 28, 2010. *brainalchemist.com/2010/07/28/15-practices-to-deepen-human-connection-and-engagement-online/.*

254 V. S. Ramachandran, "Mirror Neurons and the Brain in the Vat." *Edge: The Third Culture.* January 10, 2006. *www.edge.org/3rd_culture/ramachandran06/ramachandran06_ index.html.*

255 Michael A. Stracco, "Brain Engagement," *Brainy Bits:* "Interesting Articles," "The Brains [sic] Reaction to Cooperative Learning." *mset.rst2.edu/portfolios/s/stracco_m/ regional%20training%20courses/teaching%20brains/brain_engagement.htm.*

256 Michelle Castillo, "Study: More Friends on Facebook Equals a Bigger Amygdala in Your Brain," *Time,* December 28, 2010. *techland.time.com/2010/12/28/study-more-friends-on-facebook-equals-a-bigger-amygdala-in-your-brain/.*

257 Amanda Gardner, "Size of Key Brain Region Linked to Size of Your Social Network," *US News & World Report,* December 27, 2010. *health.usnews.com/health-news/family-health/brain-and-behavior/articles/2010/12/27/size-of-key-brain-region-linked-to-size-of-your-social-network.*

258 Aleks Krotoski, "Robin Dunbar: we can only ever have 150 friends at most …," The Observer/Guardian.co.uk, March 14, 2010. *www.guardian.co.uk/technology/2010/ mar/14/my-bright-idea-robin-dunbar.*

259 Ibid.

260 "Stayin' alive: That's what friends are for," news release from Brigham Young University, July 27, 2010. *news.byu.edu/archive10-jul-relationships.aspx.*

261 Valerie C. Crooks, et al., "Social Network, Cognitive Function, and Dementia Incidence Among Elderly Women," *American Journal of Public Health* 98, no. 7 (July 2008). *www.ncbi.nlm.nih.gov/pmc/articles/PMC2424087/.*

262 Gabrielle Selz, "Alzheimer's and the Social Cure," *Brain World,* November 1, 2010. *brainworldmagazine.com/?p=811.*

263 David A. Bennett, et al., "The effect of social networks on the relation between Alzheimer's disease pathology and level of cognitive function in old people: a longitudinal cohort study," *The Lancet Neurology* 5, no. 5 (May 2006), 406–412. *www. thelancet.com/journals/laneur/article/PIIS1474442206704173/abstract.*

264 Selz, "Alzheimer's and the Social Cure."

265 Ibid.

266 Betsy Lee, "Want a Little Instant Happy? Give a Little," *Blue Springs Journal,* November 23, 2010. *www.bluespringsjournal.com/2010/11/23/40590/want-a-little-instant-happy-give.html.*

267 Monika Guttman, "The Aging Brain," *USC Health Magazine,* Spring, 2001. *www.usc.edu/hsc/info/pr/hmm/01spring/brain.html.*

268 "How to Keep Your Brain Young and Active," eHow Health. *www.ehow.com/how_4849271_keep-brain-young-active.html#ixzz18Vi84yE3.*

269 David J. Hanson, "Drinking Alcohol, Dementia and Alzheimer's Disease," *Alcohol Problems and Solutions. www2.potsdam.edu/hansondj/HealthIssues/2007 1025202420. html.*

270 Liesi E. Hebert, et al., "Is the Risk of Developing Alzheimer's Disease Greater for Women than for Men?" *American Journal of Epidemiology* 153, no. 2 (February 15, 2000), 132–136. *aje.oxfordjournals.org/content/153/2/132.abstract.*

271 Elizabeth Arias, "United States Life Tables, 2006," *National Vital Statistics Report* 58, no. 21 (June 28, 2010), U.S. Department of Health and Human Services, Centers for Disease Control and Prevention. *www.cdc.gov/nchs/data/nvsr/nvsr58/nvsr58_21.pdf.*

272 Alzheimer's Association, "Brain Tour: Brain Basics, 5. The Neuron Forest," *Alzheimer's Association. www.alz.org/brain/05.asp.*

273 Lawrence Robinson, Joanna Saisan, and Jeanne Segal, "Signs, Symptoms, and Stages of Alzheimer's Disease," HelpGuide.org, March, 2011. *helpguide.org/elder/alzheimers_disease_symptoms_stages.htm.*

274 Ibid.

275 "Preventing Alzheimer's Disease and Cognitive Decline," final panel statement from the NIH State-of-the-Science Conference, April 26–28, 2010, NIH Consensus Development Program. *www.consensus.nih.gov/2010/alzstatement.htm.*

276 Christine Dell'Amore, "To Stave Off Alzheimer's, Learn a Language?" *National Geographic,* February 18, 2011. *news.nationalgeographic.com/news/2011/02/100218-bilingual-brains-alzheimers-dementia-science-aging/.*

277 "Brain Exercises May Slow Cognitive Decline Initially, but Speed Up Dementia Later," *Science Daily,* September 1, 2010. *www.sciencedaily.com/releases/2010/09/100901161549.htm.*

278 "About 70 percent of people have tried to meditate—Time.com," *Mediation Geek,* January 4, 2010. *www.meditationgeek.org/2010/01/about-70-percent-of-people-have-tried.html.*

279 Yi-Yuan Tang, et al., "Short-term meditation training improves attention and self-regulation," *Proceedings of the National Academy of Sciences* 104, no. 43 (October 23, 2007), 17,152–17,156. *www.pnas.org/content/104/43/17152.*

280 Gary Nixon, Brad Hagen, and Tracey Peters, "Recovery From Psychosis: A Phenomenological Inquiry," *International Journay of Mental Health and Addiction* 8, no. 4 (January 1, 2010), 620–635. *www.springerlink.com/content/h63g2673n158n839/.*

281 Barbara Bradley Hagerty, "Are Spiritual Encounters All in Your Head?" *All Things Considered,* National Public Radio, May 19, 2009. *www.npr.org/templates/story/story.php?storyId=104291534&ps=rs.*

282 Michael Speca, Linda E. Carlson, Eileen Goodey, and Maureen Angen, "A Randomized, Wait-List Controlled Clinical Trial: The Effect of a Mindfulness Meditation-Based Stress Reduction Program on Mood and Symptoms of Stress in Cancer Outpatients" *Psychosomatic Medicine* September 1, 2000, vol. 62 no. 5. 613–622.

283 Colin Allen, "The Benefits of Meditation," *Psychology Today,* April 1, 2003. *www.psychologytoday.com/articles/200304/the-benefits-meditation.*

284 These suggestions come from: Sally Kempton's *The Heart of Meditation,* Joel and Michelle Levey's *Luminous Mind,* Camille and Lorin Roche's *Meditation Made Easy,* Sharon Salzberg's *Loving-Kindness Meditation,* Joan Borysenko's *Minding the Body, Mending the Mind,* Ragini Michaels's *Facticity,* and from my own experience.

285 Patricia Carrington, "How Does Meditation Differ From Prayer?" Mastering EFT. *www.masteringeft.com/MeditationCenter/Articles/MeditationDiffersFromPrayer.htm.*

286 Newberg and Waldman.

287 Uffe Schjoedt, et al., "Highly religious participants recruit areas of social cognition in personal prayer." *Social Cognitive and Affective Neuroscience* 4, no. 2 (2009), 199–207. *scan.oxfordjournals.org/content/4/2/199.full.*

288 Newberg and Waldman.

289 Judith Heerwagen and Betty Hase, "Building Biophilia: Connecting People to Nature in Building Design," *Idaho Department of Lands: Healthy Trees, Healthy Communities, Healthy People; a Compendium of Resources on the Air, Water, Health, Energy & Economic Benefits of Community Trees,* March 8, 2001. *www.treebenefits.terrasummit.com/Documents/Health/Building%20Biophilia%20--copywrited.pdf.*

290 Ibid.

291 R. S. Ulrich, "View Through a Window May Influence Recovery from Surgery," *Science* (April, 1984) 224, 420–421.

292 Heerwagen and Hase.

293 Ibid.

294 Ibid.

295 The Prihatin Institute, "About: Research," *prihatin.org/about.html.*

296 Janet Rae-Dupree, "Can You Become a Creature of New Habits?" *The New York Times,* May 4, 2008. *www.nytimes.com/2008/05/04/business/04unbox.html.*

297 Leo Babauta, "Purpose Your Day: Most Important Task (MIT)," February 6, 2007, blog entry on ZenHabits. *zenhabits.net/purpose-your-day-most-important-task/.*

Resources

Want more information on your brain? These sources cover everything from how your brain works to how you can be more resilient in your world.

Websites

Neuroscience for Kids, explains the complexities of the brain in an accessible way:
faculty.washington.edu/chudler/neurok.html

John Ratey and the power of exercise:
johnratey.com

Team support for athletic events to support leukemia and lymphoma research:
teamintraining.com

North American Menopause Society:
menopause.org

Menopause support for baby boomers:
thirdage.com/menopause

An "activist approach" to aging:
artofaging.org

Susun Weed herbal and alternative view on menopause:
menopause-metamorphosis.com

Babeland, women-friendly sex shop:
babeland.com

Oysters and Chocolate, women-friendly erotica:
oystersandchocolate.com

About.com's sex tips for older women:
longevity.about.com/od/healthyagingandlongevity/tp/sex_tips_women.htm

Matching, logic, and word games from Set Puzzles:
setgame.com

Brain games from Parade.com:
parade.com/games/lumosity/index.html

Brain games:
lumosity.com

Tapas Acupressure Technique (TAT):
www.tatlife.com

Thought Field Therapy (developed by Roger Callahan):
www.tftrx.com

Emotional Freedom Technique (developed by Gary Craig):
www.emofree.com

Brain Injury Association:
biausa.org

Top safe cars:
topsafestcars.net

Oprah's No Phone Zone:
oprah.com/packages/no-phone-zone.html

Pollution in People's "Reading Labels to Avoid Phthalates":
pollutioninpeople.org/toxics/labels

Books

Andreasen, Nancy C. *The Creating Brain: the Neuroscience of Genius.* New York: Dana, 2005.

Becker, Gavin de. *The Gift of Fear: Survival Signals that Protect Us from Violence.* New York: Dell, 1998.

Bernstein, Carolyn. *The Migraine Brain: Your Breakthrough Guide to Fewer Headaches, Better Health.* Toronto: Simon & Schuster, 2008.

Blair, Nancy. *Thank You, Your Opinion Means Nothing to Me: A Year of Hot Flashes, Flashbacks and Finding My Voice.* London: Element, Limited, 2006.

Borysenko, Joan. *It's Not the End of the World: Developing Resilience in Times of Change.* Carlsbad, CA: Hay House, 2009.

Brown, Stuart L., and Christopher C. Vaughan. *Play: How It Shapes the Brain, Opens the Imagination, and Invigorates the Soul.* New York: Avery, 2010.

Cameron, Julia. *The Artist's Way: A Spiritual Path to Higher Creativity.* New York: Tarcher/Penguin, 2002.

Carrington, Patricia. *The Book of Meditation: the Complete Guide to Modern Meditation.* Shaftesbury, Dorset: Element, 1998.

Dement, William C., and Christopher C. Vaughan. *The Promise of Sleep: A Pioneer in Sleep Medicine Explores the Vital Connection Between Health, Happiness, and a Good Night's Sleep.* New York: Dell Trade Paperback, 2000.

Drescher, Fran. *Cancer Schmancer.* Waterville, ME: Thorndike, 2002.

Eden, Donna, and David Feinstein. *Energy Medicine.* New York: Jeremy P. Tarcher/Putnam, 1999.

Eliot, Lise. *Pink Brain, Blue Brain: How Small Differences Grow into Troublesome Gaps—and What We Can Do About It.* Boston: Houghton Mifflin Harcourt, 2009.

Fine, Cordelia. *Delusions of Gender: How Our Minds, Society, and Neurosexism Create Difference.* New York: W. W. Norton, 2010.

Gardner, Howard. *Frames of Mind: The Theory of Multiple Intelligence.* New York: Basic, 2011.

Goleman, Daniel. *Social Intelligence: The New Science of Human Relationships.* New York: Bantam, 2006.

Hallowell, Edward. *Driven to Distraction.* New York: Touchstone Press, 1995.

Katie, Byron, and Stephen Mitchell. *Loving What Is: Four Questions That Can Change Your Life.* New York: Harmony, 2002.

Kessler, David A. *The End of Overeating: Taking Control of the Insatiable American Appetite.* Emmaus, PA: Rodale, 2009.

Khalsa, Dharma Singh. *Brain Longevity: The Breakthrough Medical Program That Improves Your Mind and Memory.* New York: Grand Central Publishing, 1999.

Kornblatt, Sondra. *A Better Brain at Any Age: The Holistic Way to Improve Your Memory, Reduce Stress, and Sharpen Your Wits.* San Francisco, CA: Red Wheel/Weiser, 2008.

———. *Restful Insomnia: How to Get the Benefits of Sleep Even When You Can't.* San Francisco, CA: Red Wheel/Weiser, 2010

Legato, Marianne J., and Laura Tucker. *Why Men Never Remember and Women Never Forget.* Emmaus, PA: Rodale, 2005.

Levy, Joel and Michelle. *Luminous Mind.* San Francisco: Conari Press, 2006.

Long, Priscilla. *The Writer's Portable Mentor: a Guide to Art, Craft, and the Writing Life.* Seattle, WA: Wallingford, 2010.

Maurer, Robert. *One Small Step Can Change Your Life: The Kaizen Way.* New York: Workman, 2004.

McEwen, Bruce S., and Elizabeth Norton Lasley. *The End of Stress as We Know It.* Washington, D.C.: Joseph Henry Press, 2002.

Michaels, Ragini. *Unflappable: 6 Steps to Staying Happy, Centered, and Peaceful No Matter What.* San Francisco: Conari Press, 2012.

Nass, Clifford Ivar., and Corina Yen. *The Man Who Lied to His Laptop: What Machines Teach Us about Human Relationships.* New York: Current, 2010.

Newberg, Andrew B., and Mark Robert. Waldman. *How God Changes Your Brain: Breakthrough Findings from a Leading Neuroscientist.* New York: Ballantine Trade Paperbacks, 2010.

Northrup, Christiane. *Women's Bodies, Women's Wisdom: Creating Physical and Emotional Health and Healing.* New York: Bantam, 2006.

———. *Our Bodies, Ourselves: Menopause.* New York: Simon & Schuster, 2006.

Pearce, Joseph Chilton. *The Biology of Transcendence: A Blueprint of the Human Spirit.* Rochester, VT: Park Street, 2002.

Pert, Candace B. *Molecules of Emotion: The Science Behind Mind-Body Medicine.* New York: Scribner, 2003.

Pfaff, Donald W. *Man and Woman: An Inside Story.* New York: Oxford University Press, 2011.

Powers, William. *Hamlet's Blackberry: Building a Good Life in the Digital Age.* New York: Harper, 2010.

Ratey, John J., and Eric Hagerman. *Spark: the Revolutionary New Science of Exercise and the Brain.* New York: Little, Brown, 2008.

Ruebush, Mary. *Why Dirt Is Good: 5 Ways to Make Germs Your Friends.* New York: Kaplan, 2009.

Salzberg, Sharon. *Real Happiness: The Power of Meditation, A 28-day Program.* New York: Workman, 2011.

Shesso, Renna. *Math for Mystics: From the Fibonacci Sequence to Luna's Labyrinth to the Golden Section and Other Secrets of Sacred Geometry.* San Francisco, CA: Weiser, 2007.

Sichel, Deborah, and Jeanne Watson Driscoll. *Women's Moods , Women's Minds: What Every Woman Must Know about Hormones, the Brain, and Emotional Health.* New York: William Morrow, 1999.

Tolle, Eckhart. *The Power of Now: A Guide to Spiritual Enlightenment.* Vancouver, B.C., Canada: Namaste, 2004.

Wise, Nina. *A Big New Free Happy Unusual Life: Self-Expression and Spiritual Practice for Those Who Have Time for Neither.* New York: Broadway, 2002.

Brain Fitness for Women

Index

illness, 25–27, 62. *see also* specific illnesses
injuries, head, 70–72
inner talk, 102
insomnia, 26
intelligence, 55–56, 85
Internet, 141–146
intestines, 93
iron, 128

Jung, Carl, 66

Katz, Lawrence C., 70
Kessler, David, 107–108
Khakpour, Dori, 124
Khalsa, Dharma Singh, 119
kinesthetic learning, 84
Kraus, Nina, 81
krill oil, 114
Kumar, Channi, 44

Lafferty, Carrie, 96, 178
language training, 162
laughter, 47, 68, 88
learning
    arts training improving, 81
    exercise improving, 58, 78
    foods improving, 115, 116–117, 119
    multiple intelligences theories, 85
    play improving, 81–84
    and practice, 11–12
    styles of, 84
left *vs.* right hemispheres, 13, 86–87
Legato, Marianne J., 22
leptin, 65
light therapy, 48
limbic brain, 6, 96
longevity, 150, 159
long-term memory, 77
lupus, 26
luteinizing hormone (LH), 34–35, 35–36

magnesium, 29, 37, 40, 128
manganese, 128
mantras, 171
Mason, Paul, 95
Maurer, Robert, 182
McEwen, Bruce, 37
meats, 135
medications
    herbal remedies interacting with, 41
    hormone replacement, 33, 50–53
    migraine, 29
    postpartum depression, 48
    premenstrual pain relief, 37
    premenstrual syndrome symptoms,
        39–40

supplements interacting with, 130
meditation, 64, 102–103, 163, 166–173
melatonin, 24–25, 27
memory, 49–50, 73–80, 86, 116, 118
menopause, 24, 25, 28, 33, 48–53, 59
menstruation
    disorders associated with, 37–43
    migraines and, 28
    overview, 35–37
mercury, 134
Merzenich, Michael, 76
Michaels, Ragini, 98, 169
microalgae oils, 114
migraines, 27–29
mind-body connections, 92–95, 168–169
minerals, 29, 39, 40, 127–130
mnemonics, 79–80
monounsaturated fats, 108, 112
motorcycling, and head injuries, 72
movement, 56, 84, 94, 171. *see also* exercise
moxibustion, 42
mugwort, 42
multiple intelligences, 85
multitasking, 142–143
music, 81
myelin, 9

nail polish, 138
name memorization, 78–79, 150
nature, 174–179
neural pathways, 11
neurogenesis, 10–11, 59, 66
neurohormones, 18
neurolinguistic programming (NLP), 97
neurons
    brain anatomy and physiology, 8–11
    exercise impacting, 55, 57–58
    hormones affecting, 34
    during menopause, 50
    mirror, 148
    as pain relievers, 30
    plasticity of, 74–76
neurosexism, 14
neurotoxins. see toxins
neurotransmitters
    anxiety-reducing, 36, 58
    beverages protecting, 120
    disorders due to imbalance of, 27
    as emotional triggers, 99
    factors regulating, 39, 55, 58, 59, 68, 119
    foods guarding against depletion of, 117
    function compared to hormones, 18
    during menopause, 50
    vitamins supporting, 126
Newberg, Andrew, 67, 167, 173, 174
Nhat Han, Thich, 69

About the Author

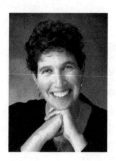

SONDRA KORNBLATT is a health writer and developer of the Restful Insomnia program, which helps people rest when they can't sleep. She is the author of *A Better Brain at Any Age* and *Restful Insomnia*, both published by Conari Press. She and her family live in the Seattle area. Learn more at www.brainfitnessforwomen.com.

To Our Readers